CRITICAL CARE CLINICS

Terrorism and Critical Care:
Chemical, Biologic, Radiologic,
and Nuclear Weapons

GUEST EDITORS
Jerris R. Hedges, MD, MS
Robert G. Hendrickson, MD

CONSULTING EDITORS
Richard W. Carlson, MD, PhD
Michael A. Geheb, MD

October 2005 • Volume 21 • Number 4

SAUNDERS

An Imprint of Elsevier, Inc.
PHILADELPHIA LONDON TORONTO MONTREAL SYDNEY TOKYO

W.B. SAUNDERS COMPANY
A Division of Elsevier Inc.

Elsevier Inc. • 1600 John F. Kennedy Blvd., Suite 1800 • Philadelphia, Pennsylvania 19103-2899

http://www.theclinics.com

CRITICAL CARE CLINICS Volume 21, Number 4
October 2005 ISSN 0749-0704
Editor: Joe Rusko ISBN 1-4160-2685-1

Reprints. For copies of 100 or more, of articles in this publication, please contact the Commercial Reprints Department, Elsevier Inc., 360 Park Avenue South, New York, New York 10010-1710. Phone: (212) 633-3813; Fax: (212) 462-1935; E-mail: reprints@elsevier.com

The ideas and opinions expressed in *Critical Care Clinics* do not necessarily reflect those of the Publisher. The Publisher does not assume any responsibility for any injury and/or damage to persons or property arising out of or related to any use of the material contained in this periodical. The reader is advised to check the appropriate medical literature and the product information currently provided by the manufacturer of each drug to be administered to verify the dosage, the method and duration of administration, or contraindications. It is the responsibility of the treating physician or other health care professional, relying on independent experience and knowledge of the patient, to determine drug dosages and the best treatment for the patient. Mention of any product in this issue should not be construed as endorsement by the contributors, editors, or the Publisher of the product or manufacturers' claims.

Critical Care Clinics (ISSN 0749-0704) is published quarterly by W.B. Saunders Company. Corporate and editorial offices: Elsevier Inc., 1600 John F. Kennedy Blvd., Philadelphia, PA 19103-2899. Accounting and circulation offices: 6277 Sea Harbor Drive, Orlando, FL 32887-4800. Periodicals postage paid at Orlando, FL 32862, and additional mailing offices. Subscription prices are $170.00 per year for US individuals, $280.00 per year for US institution, $85.00 per year for US students and residents, $210.00 per year for Canadian individuals, $340.00 per year for Canadian institutions, $230.00 per year for international individuals, $340.00 per year for international institutions and $115.00 per year for Canadian and foreign students/residents. To receive student/resident rate, orders must be accompanied by name of affiliated institution, date of term, and the *signature* of program/residency coordinator on institution letterhead. Orders will be billed at individual rate until proof of status is received. Foreign air speed delivery is included in all *Clinics* subscription prices. All prices are subject to change without notice. POSTMASTER: Send address changes to *Critical Care Clinics*, W.B. Saunders Company, Periodicals Fulfillment, Orlando, FL 32887-4800. **Customer Service: 1-800-654-2452 (US). From outside of the US, call 1-407-345-1000. E-mail: hhspcs@harcourt.com**

Critical Care Clinics is also published in Spanish by Editorial Inter-Medica, Junin 917, 1er A, 1113, Buenos Aires, Argentina.

Critical Care Clinics is covered in *Index Medicus, EMBASE/Excerpta Medica, Current Concepts/ Clinical Medicine, ISI/BIOMED,* and *Chemical Abstracts.*

Printed in the United States of America.

CONSULTING EDITORS

RICHARD W. CARLSON, MD, PhD, Chairman, Department of Internal Medicine, Marcopia Medical Center; and Professor, Department of Medicine, Mayo Graduate School of Medicine, Phoenix Arizona

MICHAEL A. GEHEB, MD, Professor, Department of Medicine, and Vice President, Clinical Programs, Oregon Health & Science University, Portland, Oregon

GUEST EDITORS

JERRIS R. HEDGES, MD, MS, Professor of Emergency Medicine, Chairman, Department of Emergency Medicine; Chief, Emergency Services, Oregon Health & Science University, Portland, Oregon

ROBERT G. HENDRICKSON, MD, Assistant Professor, Department of Emergency Medicine, Oregon Health & Science University, Portland; Medical Toxicologist, Oregon Poison Center, Portland, Oregon

CONTRIBUTORS

CLAUDIA L. BARTHOLD, MD, Fellow in Medical Toxicology, Georgia Poison Center, Emory University School of Medicine, Atlanta, Georgia

JOHN W. BURNHAM, PhD, Director, Environmental Health and Radiation Safety, Oregon Health & Science University, Portland, Oregon

MOHAMUD DAYA, MD, MS, Associate Professor, Department of Emergency Medicine, Oregon Health & Science University, Portland, Oregon

JANET FRANCO, MS, Clinical Radiation Safety Officer, Environmental Health and Radiation Safety, Oregon Health & Science University, Portland, Oregon

ROBERT G. HENDRICKSON, MD, Assistant Professor, Department of Emergency Medicine, Oregon Health & Science University, Portland; Medical Toxicologist, Oregon Poison Center, Portland, Oregon

JERRIS R. HEDGES, MD, MS, Professor of Emergency Medicine, Chairman, Department of Emergency Medicine; Chief, Emergency Services, Oregon Health & Science University, Portland, Oregon

B. ZANE HOROWITZ, MD, FACMT, Professor of Emergency Medicine, Oregon Health & Science University, Portland; Medical Director, Oregon Poison Center, Portland, Oregon

MARC HOUSTON, DO, Instructor of Emergency Medicine, Fellow, Emergency Medical Services, Oregon Health & Science University, Portland, Oregon

KERMIT HUEBNER, MD, US Army Medical Research Institute of Infectious Diseases, Fort Detrick, Maryland

JOHN McMANUS, MD, MCR, FACEP, Research Physician, US Army Research Program for Combat Casualty Care, US Army Institute of Surgical Research, Transitional Program Director, San Antonio Uniformed Services Health Education Consortium, Fort Sam Houston, Texas; Adjunct Assistant Professor, Department of Emergency Medicine, Oregon Health & Science University, Portland, Oregon; Uniformed Services University of Health Sciences, Bethesda, Maryland

ANTHONY P. MOROCCO, MD, Clinical Assistant Professor, Department of Emergency Medicine, Oregon Health & Science University School of Medicine; Chairman and Medical Toxicologist, Department of Emergency Medicine, Guam Memorial Hospital, Oka Tamuning; and Medical Director, Emergency Medical Services, Guam Department of Public Health and Social Services, Mangilao, Guam

SARAH D. NAFZIGER, MD, Assistant Professor, Department of Emergency Medicine, Associate Scientist, Center for Emergency Care and Disaster Preparedness, University of Alabama at Burmingham, Birmingham, Alabama

YOKO NAKAMURA, MD, Visiting Physician, Department of Emergency Medicine, Oregon Health & Science University, Portland, Oregon

DAVID C. PIGOTT, MD, Associate Professor of Emergency Medicine, Department of Emergency Medicine, The University of Alabama at Birmingham, Birmingham, Alabama

JOSHUA G. SCHIER, MD, Assistant Professor of Emergency Medicine, Emory University School of Medicine, Atlanta, Georgia

LAURA SPIVAK, MD, Medical Toxicology Fellow, Oregon Poison Control Center, Portland; Instructor, Department of Emergency Medicine, Oregon Health & Science University, Portland, Oregon

CRAIG R. WARDEN, MD, MPH, Associate Professor, Emergency Medicine and Pediatrics, Oregon Health & Science University, Portland; Attending Medical Toxicologist, Oregon Regional Poison Center; Medical Director, Clackamas County Fire District # 1, Portland, Oregon

CONTENTS

depend on the affinity of the OPC for muscarinic versus nicotinic receptors, and are likely to include both. Muscarinic symptoms may include diarrhea, urination, bronchospasm, bronchorrhea, emesis, and salivation. Nicotinic symptoms such as paralysis and fasciculations may also occur. Central nervous system toxicity may include seizures, altered mental status, and apnea, and require prompt intervention. Treatment includes early airway and ventilatory support as well as antidotal therapy with atropine, pralidoxime, and diazepam. Goals of therapy include prevention and rapid treatment of hypoxia and seizures, as these are linked to patient outcome.

Cyanides

Anthony P. Morocco

Cyanide is a likely weapon for terrorists due to its notoriety, lethality, and availability. Poisoning results in central nervous system and cardiovascular dysfunction due to inhibition of oxidative phosphorylation. Laboratory findings of anion gap metabolic acidosis and hyperlactemia aid in confirming the diagnosis. Treatment for significant poisonings includes aggressive supportive care and administration of antidotes such as sodium nitrite, sodium thiosulfate, and hydroxocobalamin. Survivors of significant poisonings can have long-term neurologic dysfunction.

John McManus and Kermit Huebner

Vesicants (or blister agents) are cytotoxic alkylating compounds, which are chemical agents sometimes collectively known as mustard gas or simply as mustard. Other blister agents are nitrogen mustard; sulfur mustard; lewisite, a vesicant that contains arsenic; and phosgene oxime, a halogenated oxime that possesses different properties and toxicity from the other agents. This article discusses history, toxicity, clinical presentation, and common treatment for vesicants.

Craig R. Warden

There are many chemical respiratory agents suitable for use by terrorists. They are the oldest chemical agents used and have caused the most casualties throughout the 20th century. Many are available in large quantities for industrial use and are susceptible to potential sabotage. This paper will concentrate on respiratory agents that are readily available and have the potential to cause a large number of casualties and panic. These agents have a lower rate of lethality when compared to other chemical agents but could produce many casualties that may overwhelm the emergency medical system.

medicine and critical care physicians are familiar with the care and treatment of an accidentally or intentionally irradiated patient who is contaminated externally or internally. This article reviews basic radiobiology and the variety of clinical signs and symptoms exhibited by victims exposed to radiation. Preparation for patient receipt and emergency care, followed by definitive diagnosis using biodosimetry is also presented. Therapeutic measures continue to evolve for externally and internally exposed victims, including those with combined injuries caused by burns and trauma.

Ricin is a potent toxin found within the beans of the castor plant. Ricin's widespread availability makes it a viable biological weapon. Ricin intoxication mimics a variety of disease states, thus a low threshold of suspicion must be maintained to recognize a potential epidemic. Treatment is largely supportive.

Botulinum toxin is regarded as the most lethal substance known. It is estimated that the human LD_{50} for inhalation botulism is 1 to 3 nanograms of toxin/kilogram body mass. Although only three cases of inhalational botulism have been described, an understanding of the pathophysiology of food-borne outbreaks, wound botulism, and infant botulism, and their therapies, enables the medical community to plan treatment in the event of an aerosol release of botulinum toxin. Antitoxin, vaccine, and $F(ab')_2$ immune fragment therapies are discussed as adjuncts to supportive therapy.

FORTHCOMING ISSUES

RECENT ISSUES

ELSEVIER
SAUNDERS

Crit Care Clin 21 (2005) 641–652

CRITICAL
CARE
CLINICS

Introduction—What Critical Care Practitioners Should Know About Terrorism Agents

Robert G. Hendrickson, MD*, Jerris R. Hedges, MD, MS

Department of Emergency Medicine, Oregon Health and Science University, Oregon Poison Center, 3181 S.W. Sam Jackson Park Road, CBS 550, Portland, OR 97201-3098, USA

Terrorist attack is a prime concern of local and national emergency planners. Since 2001, much work has been done to enhance critical infrastructure and training for first responders; however, the preparation of health care practitioners to recognize, diagnose, and treat the victims of terrorist events remains a major hurdle. Although it is not possible for health care practitioners to know every detail of every possible scenario, agent, and illness, some scenarios or agents are seen as more likely agents of terror. This edition reviews the diagnosis, testing, and treatment of the most likely biologic, radiologic, and chemical agents likely to be used by terrorists.

The information provided concentrates on the critical care aspects of these diseases and agents. Other health-care providers and administrators may look upon critical care professionals for guidance in the setting of a terrorist attack. For that reason, some information on decontamination, personal protective equipment, and antidotes will be given for completeness, even though they are likely to be used before the patient arriving at the critical care unit.

In preparing for future terrorist attacks, it is important to review the past military and terrorist uses of these agents to discuss ways in which critical care professionals can prepare for such events.

Brief history of chemical, biologic, radiologic, and nuclear weapons in warfare

The use of chemicals and infectious agents to gain advantage during warfare dates back many centuries. Radioisotope and nuclear weapons use is, of course, a

* Corresponding author.
E-mail address: hendriro@ohsu.edu (R.G. Hendrickson).

doi:10.1016/j.ccc.2005.05.009
criticalcare.theclinics.com

more recent invention. Many agents, including chemical, biologic, and radio-logic, have been significantly studied by several of the world militaries for use in warfare. The specifics of the most effective dosing, release characteristics, environmental conditions, and delivery have been perfected for many of these military agents. A review of the uses, and the effect, of these agents during warfare is helpful in preparing for modern events, because these agents remain some of the most likely agents to be used by terrorists.

Chemical agents

Chemical agents are chemicals that may be used by terrorists or militaries with the aim of producing mass casualties and terror [1]. These agents include those that were specifically designed by military agencies (eg, sarin, VX, mustard, and so on), as well as chemicals that are routinely used in industrial processes (eg, chlorine, phosgene, ammonia, cyanide, and so on).

Chemicals have been used in warfare for many centuries. Early examples of chemical warfare mostly include the burning of chemicals to produce noxious smoke clouds. The Chinese created noxious arsenic smokes in warfare as early as 1000 BC [2]. In 423 BC, the Spartans created sulfur dioxide by burning coal, sulfur, and pitch, and directed the smoke into forts held by Athenian forces during the Pelopennesian War [2]. Leonardo daVinci proposed the dispersal of sulfide of arsenic and verdigris (copper acetates) against invading ships in the fifteenth century [2]. In more modern times, chemical warfare planning became more advanced. In the nineteenth century, chemists and military planners in Great Britain, the United States, and France, conceived of weaponry to deploy cacodyl cyanide, chlorine, and bromoacetate, respectively [2].

However, in April 1915, the first large-scale use of a chemical agent in warfare occurred in Ypres, Belgium, when German forces released over 150 tons of chlorine gas against French and Canadian troops [3]. This release sparked an explosion of chemical military attacks throughout World War I (WWI). During this war, chemical casualties made up 2% to 4.5% of casualties to German, French, British, Russian, and United States troops, totaling 690,000 casualties [2]. By the end of the war, up to 25% of all artillery shells contained chemical agents [2], and over 100,000 tons of chemical agents had been used by Great Britain (chlorine), France (cyanide, cyanogen chloride), and Germany (chlorine, phosgene, diphosgene, mustard, chloropicrin) [4].

Following WWI, growing concerns over the use of chemical weapons led to the drafting of the Geneva Protocol (1925), which condemned the offensive initial use of chemical agents. The Protocol was signed and ratified by many of the world's nations, including those that would go on to manufacture, store, and use chemical agents years later. The United States signed the Protocol; however, Congress refused to ratify it (it was eventually ratified in 1974 and signed by the President in 1975).

Although no chemical agents were used in warfare during World War II (WWII), production was at an all time high. During the war, Germany produced over 2000 tons of mustard, 30,000 tons of tabun, and 500 tons of sarin [5], Japan produced over 8000 tons of mustard, Lewisite, and hydrogen cyanide [2], and the United States produced 20,000 tons of phosgene, 87,000 tons of mustard, 20,000 tons of Lewisite, 12,500 tons of cyanogen chloride, and 560 tons of hydrogen cyanide [2].

In the years up to and after WWII, several of the world's militaries intensively researched a variety of chemicals and dispersal techniques. Additional chemical agents were added to military arsenals including tabun (synthesized 1936, military production 1942), sarin (synthesized 1937, military production 1942), soman (synthesized 1944), VX (synthesized 1950) [2], and 3-quinuclidynl benzilate (BZ) (synthesized in 1962) [2,5]. In addition, advanced delivery techniques were developed to make targeted attacks possible [1]. The United States (through the Chemical Warfare Service) and the Soviet Union continued to research and refine their chemical weapons. Additional nations acquired or used offensive chemical weapons during this time, including the Balkan states, Bulgaria, Burma, China, Czechoslovakia, Egypt, Ethiopia, France, Hungary, Indonesia, Iran, Iraq, Israel, Laos, Libya, North Korea, Romania, South Africa, Syria, Taiwan, and Vietnam [6].

Several significant uses of chemical agents occurred during this time. In 1967, Egyptian airplanes dropped bombs filled with mustard and nerve agent on the Yemeni villages of Kitaf, Gahar, Gabas, Hofal, Gadr, and Gadafa, killing at least 500 people [2]. Chemical agents were again used during the Iran–Iraq war between 1983 and 1988 [7]. Iraq mostly used airplanes to deliver mustard agent, cyanides, and the nerve agents tabun and sarin [7]. Up to 5% of Iranian casualties were due to chemical agent injuries during this war. In the same time period, both the United States and the Soviet Union began to destroy their existing stockpiles of chemical weapons. However, Iraq continued to produce chemical agents, and at the end of the 1991 Gulf War, Iraq was maintaining stockpiles of mustard agent, botulinum toxin, and the nerve agents tabun and sarin [5,8].

Biologic agents

Biologic agents are those agents that are, or are derived from, living organisms that may be used by terrorists or militaries with the aim of producing mass casualties and terror. These agents include viruses, bacteria, and bacterial or plant toxins.

Biologic agents have been used in warfare for centuries. Their early use involved largely exposing opposing troops to infected bodies or animals. In 1346, the Tartars hurled the cadavers of people who had died of the plague into the city of Caffa, producing a retreat of those forces [2,9,10]. Similarly, in 1710, the Russians hurled plague-infected bodies into Swedish-held Reval, Estonia [2,9]. In 1650, a Polish general placed the saliva of rabid dogs into artillery for firing against his enemies [2]. The British used a somewhat different technique during the Pontiac's Rebellion in New England in 1763. British soldiers distributed blankets from smallpox-infected patients to the Native American population, who had little immunity to the disease [10]. It is estimated that half of the tribal population died as a result [11].

Additional uses of biologic agents continued until WWI. During this war, despite several nations developing and deploying biologic weaponry, there was no major release of any agent. However, there were several cases of biologic tampering with livestock. In one case, undercover German operatives attempted to infect horses and mules in the United States with the bacteria that causes glanders (*Pseudomonas pseudomallei*). The horses and mules were bound for the western front, and were to be used by Allied forces. Several other unsubstantiated reports exist of German forces attempting to spread plague, cholera, and glanders [9,10].

After the 1930s, the development and production of biologic agents by the United States Biologic Weapons Program, the Soviet Biopreparat program, France, Canada, Great Britain, Japan, and Germany continued. The Japanese had a particularly advanced biologic weapons program run by their Imperial Unit 731. The Japanese were able to develop weaponry and to disperse typhus, rickettsia, anthrax, and cholera against Chinese civilians and troops [9]. They also developed a system to infect fleas with plague and drop them upon Ning Bo, a village in China. This release reportedly led to 500 plague deaths in the village [2]. Unit 731 performed numerous experiments on thousands of prisoners of WWII, leading to over 1000 prisoner deaths from anthrax, botulism, brucellosis, cholera, Shigella, Salmonella, meningococcemia, and plague [9,10].

Although the Biologic Weapons Convention (BWC) was signed in 1972, several nations continued their production of biologic weapons, including the Soviet Union and Iraq [9]. Nine years after signing the BWC, anthrax was unintentionally released from a processing plant in Sverdlosk in the Soviet Union. The anthrax spores were released as an aerosol in an urban center, and led to the development of anthrax in 96 people and caused 64 deaths [12]. When the Soviet Union collapsed in 1991, concerns arose about the security of the biologic weapons of the former Soviet states [13]. Reports of poor or no security at military instillations and military laboratories suggest that agents (eg, botulinum toxin, anthrax, and smallpox) and technology may have been lost to nonmilitary personnel or agencies [11,13]. In addition, concerns remain that several countries continue to research biologic agents [10].

In the following few years, it became evident that Iraq had been developing, producing, and stockpiling significant amounts of biologic weapons. Before the Persian Gulf War, Iraq had produced 125,000 gallons of biologic agent that included anthrax, aflatoxin B, and at least 19,000 L of botulinum toxin [8]. Iraq later admitted to having over 200 biologic missiles and bombs prepared during the war [2], including 100 bombs containing botulinum toxin, 50 containing anthrax spores, and 7 containing aflatoxin [14].

Radiologic agents

Radiologic agents are methods of distributing radioisotope in a manner that will affect people or disrupt normal functioning in a region. The most simple, and the most likely, way of distributing radioisotope is to combine the isotope within a conventional weapon [15]. This arrangement has commonly been referred to as a "dirty bomb" or a radiologic dispersal device. "Dirty bombs" do more to spread terror and cause traumatic injuries than actually inflict radiation-related damage [16], so they have not been used by militaries in warfare. However, several nations have researched these weapons.

Iraq reportedly experimented with "dirty bomb" technology during the 1990s. It is reported that they were unable to develop a weapon that distributed radio-isotope in a way that would produce toxicity. The United States also researched this type of weaponry, but likely for similar reasons, abandoned that program.

Nuclear weapons

Military interest in producing a nuclear weapon began shortly after the 1939 discovery of nuclear fission by German scientists Hahn and Strassman. Through the work of the "Manhattan Project," the world's first nuclear weapon ("Trinity") was detonated in New Mexico on July 16, 1945.

Several months later, on August 5, 1945, a 15-kiloton nuclear weapon ("Little Boy") was dropped on Hiroshima, Japan. Four days later, a 23-kiloton weapon ("Fat Man") was detonated over Nagasaki, Japan. It is estimated that both of these weapons produced approximately 200,000 deaths each.

Since that time, nuclear technology has progressed. Several former members of the Soviet government have reported that small, light, 0.5 to 1.0 kilotons (the explosive power of 500 to 1000 pounds of TNT) nuclear weapons have been produced ("suitcase bombs"), and can be transported and detonated by a single person [17]. Several hundred of these weapons may have been produced by the Soviet Union, the United States, and other nations. After the fall of the Soviet Union, there have been questions as to the whereabouts of many of these portable nuclear devices [17]. There is additional speculation, although certainly not definitive, that Al Queda has attempted to purchase these weapons as well.

Over the last 60 years, many nations have developed or been sold nuclear technology. The United States and the Russian Federation currently deploy approximately 10,000 warheads each, and have an agreement (the Strategic Offensive Reductions Treaty) to reduce that number to 2200 by 2012. Great Britain, Israel, and France have approximately 200, 200, and 400 warheads, respectively. China, Pakistan, and India have warhead stockpiles in the 10 to 40 range.

Nations with nuclear weapons

China
India
Israel
France
Pakistan
Russian Federation

United Kingdom
United States

Past chemical, biologic, radiologic, or nuclear agents use by terrorists

Until the previous few decades, chemical, biologic, radiologic, or nuclear agents (CBRN) were developed and produced only by nation-states. Due to significant research and development by these nations, increases in technology, and increased size and funding for terrorist groups, the use of CBRN agents by terrorist organizations has become a major concern. To better understand the potential future uses of CBRN agents by terrorists, it is important to review the previous uses by these groups.

There are significant differences in the characteristics of CBRN weapons and releases between terrorist uses and military uses. When used in military campaigns, the ideal characteristics of a CBRN weapon are agents that produce the rapid and large-scale incapacitation of troops. Military weapons may be designed to rapidly evaporate, thereby allowing friendly troops to travel through the area, or to be persistent in the environment, allowing that area to be temporarily uninhabitable. Finally, military agents may be delivered in large volumes over large distances by mortar, rocket, or bomb.

Conversely, terrorist groups may choose agents that produce large-scale fear, panic, and terror, as opposed to death or incapacitation. Terrorist attacks may be targeted at more specific populations and events or buildings with financial or political meaning. Terrorist groups may choose to use smaller volumes of agent to escape detection [1] and to produce large numbers of fearful citizens that overwhelm the health care, financial, and security systems of the region. Finally, terrorist organizations may choose to use agents that are readily available in large quantities, such as storage or transport facilities of industrial chemicals (eg, chlorine).

Chemical agent releases by terrorist organizations

There are several examples of terrorist organizations releasing chemical agents in civilian populations. In 1994, an organization named Aum Shinrikyo, released the nerve agent sarin in a residential area of the city of Matsumoto, Japan. The organization was attempting to target a group of judges who they felt were poised to make a ruling that was unfavorable to them. They produced liquid sarin and fitted a refrigeration truck with metal tanks, a heater, and fan. The liquid sarin was heated, vaporized, and directed out of the van toward the apartment building where these judges were located. This fairly low-tech release of sarin produced 600 victims, of whom 58 were hospitalized, and 7 died [18].

One year later, the same organization again used sarin on civilians. This time the group targeted the Japanese National Government's ministry offices in Tokyo, Japan. Liquid sarin was contained in plastic bags and wrapped with newspaper. Aum Shinrikyo members entered five different subways, placed the bags under the subway seats, and pierced them with the sharpened end of an umbrella to release the liquid [19]. The liquid then evaporated as the five cars approached the subway station that was directly below the ministry offices. Following the event, over 5000 people sought care related to the event, and 12 died [19]. One Tokyo hospital received 640 patients related to the release in the first day, including 111 admitted patients, 5 patients requiring mechanical ventilation, and 2 deaths [19,20].

In 1984, the world's worst industrial disaster occurred in Bhopal, India. There has been considerable controversy over whether this event was an industrial accident or the intentional actions of individuals. Whether or not it was an intentional event, Bhopal is an example of the potential effectiveness of the large-scale release of chemical agents. During the night of December 2, approximately 27 metric tons methyl isocyanate, and possibly hydrogen cyanide, phosgene, carbon monoxide, and nitrogen oxides were released in a highly populated area [21]. The release exposed 200,000 residents, producing 80,000 victims and 3000 deaths [22].

Biologic agent releases by terrorist organizations

Several examples of the production and release of biologic agents against civilians exist. In 1984, a group of followers of the Indian guru Bhagwan Shree Rajneesh attempted to affect the results of a local election that they felt would alter decisions on land use on their property. The group obtained a strain of *Salmonella typhimurium* from a commercial supplier and contaminated salad bars and coffee creamers in several restaurants in The Dalles, Oregon. Their contamination led to diarrheal illness in 751 people and 45 hospitalizations [10,23].

Aum Shinrikyo, the religious organization responsible for the sarin releases in Tokyo and Matsumoto, Japan, also researched biologic agents, including botulinum toxin and anthrax. In 1993, the group aerosolized a liquid suspension of *Bacillus anthracis* on the roof of their headquarters in Kameido, Japan [24]. No casualties were reported because the strain that was released (Sterne 34F2 strain) is intended for veterinary vaccination, and does not cause clinical anthrax [24]. Aum Shinrikyo likely released anthrax several additional times [25], and may have also released *Clostridium botulinum* aerosols at least three times in Tokyo, Japan, as well as at United States military instillations in Japan [14].

Anthrax was, of course, also dispersed via the mail in the United States in 2001. At least five letters that contained anthrax spores were sent from Trenton, New Jersey, to locations in Washington, DC, Florida, and New York, resulting in 11 inhalational and 11 cutaneous anthrax cases and five deaths [25].

Radiologic and nuclear use by terrorists

There have been no reported uses of radioisotopes in "dirty bombs" or nuclear weapon use by terrorists. However, given the ubiquity of radioisotopes used in energy production, industry, and in medicine, as well as the uncertainty about the location of Soviet nuclear weaponry, "dirty bombs" and low-yield mobile nuclear weapons remain a concern.

Likely agents given available technology, world travel, and past terrorist events

Health care practitioners cannot possibly be prepared for every possible chemical, biologic/infectious, or radiologic/nuclear event. Preparedness must concentrate on those events that are most likely to occur. To determine which events are the most likely, we must first explore the characteristics, technology, and availability of agents that make them attractive to terrorists as well as intelligence sources and known seizures of agents from terrorist groups.

Chemical agents

For a chemical release to produce large numbers of critically ill casualties, the release would likely require either a chemical released within an enclosed space or a very large volume of chemical released close to a population center [1]. As there are logistic barriers to the production and transport of a large volume of chemical agent, the most likely terrorist event is the release of a large volume of an industrial chemical that is either stored near a population center or in transit (eg, rail or truck). An alternative scenario may be a release of a small volume of aerosol or vapor into an air-handling system of a stadium or gathering place or the addition of a chemical to a local water supply.

Chemical characteristics that are ideal for terrorist agents include those chemicals that can be made into an aerosol or vapor (or evaporate readily), are liquid at room temperature (for ease of transport), and are available and stored in large quantities near population centers. Several agents fit these criteria, and include chlorine and ammonia, as well as phosgene, isocyanates, cyanides, and acids/bases. Several of these agents are consistently the most common chemicals identified in unintentional hazardous materials releases [26–28]. This reflects how commonly they are used in industry in the United States, and how commonly they are found in transport and storage near population centers.

Other chemicals of high risk include those where a significant amount of military research and development has been spent on fine-tuning delivery systems and production. Agents that have name recognition by the general population may also be seen as more effective in producing fear and panic by terrorist organizations (eg, sarin). These military agents include the vesicants (lewisite, mustard, and so on) and nerve agents (sarin, tabun, soman, VX, and so on).

Biologic agents

Release of an infectious/biologic agent may occur in several ways. A biologic agent may be released into the air as a vapor or aerosol. This method has been studied by the Soviet Union, Iraq, and the United States [25], as well as the

Aum Shinrikyo [24]. In fact, a 1970 World Health Organization study estimated that the release of 50 kg of *B anthracis* over a population center of 5 million would produce 100,000 deaths [25]. Biologic agents may also be introduced into the food or water supply, as occurred in The Dalles, Oregon, in 1984 [23]. Alternatively, a highly infectious agent can be distributed via mail or other distribution method. Finally, given the ability to rapidly fly via airplane to multiple destinations within a short period, a person who is infected with a highly contagious biologic agent (eg, viral hemorrhagic fever) could travel extensively during the contagious period and infect citizens worldwide.

Characteristics that make certain biologic agents more likely agents of terror include those that can either be released easily or are highly contagious. Release of a biologic agent requires that the agent can be produced to form an aerosol of small particles and can withstand environmental stresses (eg, anthrax spores, ricin, botulinum toxin). A significant amount of technology and expertise is required to produce a highly effective aerosolizable biologic agent that is easy to disseminate, and forms a range of vapor droplet size that make it highly effective. However, a much lesser amount of expertise would be required to produce a large volume of less-effective biologic agent that could produce casualties and widespread fear [29]. Alternatively, a biologic agent may be effective if it is highly contagious, transmittable through respiratory droplets, and there is a lack of population immunity (eg, smallpox). Agents fitting this description could be spread extensively via one or a small group of infected individuals.

Given the above characteristics, the small list of potential biologic agents mostly includes those agents where much research and development has been expended to perfect delivery. These agents include smallpox, anthrax, plague, tularemia, the hemorrhagic viruses, botulinum toxin, and ricin.

Radiologic agents

Deployment of a radiologic agent is likely to occur in one of three ways. Inclusion of commonly available radioisotopes into a conventional explosive device ("dirty bomb") is the most likely event. Radioisotopes might also be used as a "simple radiologic device" where a beta- or gamma-emitting radioisotope is positioned to expose individuals to radiation; however, this would be a highly ineffective method, and is not likely. Finally, the manipulation of nuclear facilities may be attempted to produce an explosion that releases radioisotopes.

The main characteristic of a radioisotope that would be used in a terrorist event is that it is readily available. Other issues, including the type of radiation that it emits (eg, alpha, beta, gamma) and its half-life do effect its efficacy. However, the purpose of a "dirty bomb" or other radiologic device is to produce fear and to disrupt functionality of the local region, not to produce radiation casualties. Given this, radiation type and half-life are likely of lesser importance in choosing a radioisotope. Radioisotopes are readily available in the medical field (eg, Iodine-131, Technetium-99, Cesium-137) and in industry (eg, Iridium-192, Strontium-90) where they are used to x-ray ship welds, determine flow speeds in pipes, irradiate food, and many other uses. Likely, radioisotopes include Iodine-131, Cobalt-60, Cesium-137, Americium-241, Strontium-90, and Uranium (235 or 238).

Role of poison center, public health, and federal agencies in terrorist events

Many of the resources that may assist the critical care professional in the event of a disaster are agencies that are not commonly contacted. Agencies such as the local and state public health agency, the regional Poison Control Center, Department of Homeland Security, the Centers for Disease Control and Prevention (CDC), the Federal Bureau of Investigations (FBI), the Occupational Safety and Health Administration, and the state or regional public health laboratory will all be coordinating information sharing and responses during a disaster, and may either request assistance from, or extend assistance to, critical care professionals. It is important to note that these agencies may notify hospitals and critical care practitioners of potential impending events (eg, FBI, CDC, Poison Control Center), and may be able to assist in diagnosing, decontaminating, and treating patients with unfamiliar diseases or exposures (eg, Poison Control Center).

Regional Poison Control Centers throughout the country participate in a syndromic surveillance system that may help to identify covert chemical or biologic agent releases. Every few minutes, patient information from every Poison Control Center in the country is downloaded to a central database at the American Association of Poison Control Centers in Washington, DC. The data are analyzed in real time to determine spikes in unusual diseases, unusual combinations of symptoms (eg, "food poisoning" and "hypotension"), or increases in call volume or symptom volume. In this way, Poison Control Centers hope to identify covert activity early and communicate with the health care community about identifying cases, diagnosis, antidotal therapy, and treatment of covert terrorist releases.

The regional Poison Control Center and public health agencies may also be able to serve as a resource of reliable information on agents that are not commonly seen in intensive care units. The Poison Control Center should serve as a resource to intensive care professionals on identifying terrorist agents, as well as advice on decontamination techniques and personal protective equipment, and information on diagnostic testing and treatment modalities (antibiotics/antidotes). The Poison Control Center and the public health agencies may also be able to identify antidotes that are available in area hospitals or regional caches.

Local and state public health agencies may also assist in the location of area antidotes or antibiotics. Public health agencies and regional laboratories may assist in determining appropriate testing for exposed patients, how to package, and where to send patient specimens.

State, regional, and local resources may become available in a disaster to replenish and supply antidotes, antibiotics, other pharmaceuticals, ventilators, and supplies. Critical care professionals should familiarize themselves with the available caches in their areas. The Strategic National Stockpile is a federal cache that may be deployed in a large disaster and may be available within 12 hours of activation. The Strategic National Stockpile stockpile includes basic supplies, pharmaceuticals, and ventilators.

How critical care practitioners can become prepared

Critical care professionals should be active participants in the emergency preparedness process in their hospitals. They should become familiar with the hospital emergency preparedness plan and, more importantly, with the players involved with emergency preparedness at their institution. Critical care professionals should participate in local exercises and become familiar with the methods of decontamination and the emergency plan of the hospital emergency department.

Additional planning should be undertaken to prepare the intensive care unit for terrorist events. A plan to care for additional patients over the typical intensive care unit occupancy ("surge capacity") should be put in place. Additional consideration of the need for negative pressure rooms, staff personal protective equipment for highly contagious biologic agents (eg, viral hemorrhagic fever), isolation, and decontamination should be addressed. In addition, plans to enhance staffing and potentially use volunteer health care workers to manage less severely ill patients should be explored [30].

In the event of a disaster, emergency department and intensive care unit staff members will be consulted for guidance by hospital staff and administration. This edition of the Clinics will extend the knowledge of the critical care professional on a variety of potential terrorist agents, and also help stimulate disaster planning within the critical care community.

References

[1] Hendrickson RG. Terrorist chemical releases: assessment of medical risk and implications for emergency preparedness. Hum Ecol Risk Assessment 2005;11(3):1–13.

[2] Smart JK. History of chemical and biological warfare: an American perspective. In: Sidell FR, Takafuji ET, Franz DR, editors. Textbook of military medicine: medical aspects of chemical and biological warfare. Washington (DC): Office of The Surgeon General at TMM Publications; 1997. p. 9–86.

[3] Trumpener U. The road to Ypres: the beginnings of gas warfare in World War I. J Mod Hist 1975;47:460–80.

[4] Joy RJ. Historical aspects of medical defense against chemical warfare. In: Sidell FR, Takafuji ET, Franz DR, editors. Medical aspects of chemical and biological warfare. Washington (DC): Office of the Surgeon General at TMM publications; 1997. p. 87–110.

[5] Sidell FR, Borak J. Chemical warfare agents: II. Nerve agents. Ann Emerg Med 1992;21: 865–71.

[6] Takafuji ET, Kok AB. The chemical warfare threat and the military healthcare provider. In: Sidell FR, Takafuji ET, Franz DR, editors. Textbook of military medicine: medical aspects of chemical and biological warfare. Washington (DC): Office of The Surgeon General at TMM Publications; 1997. p. 111–28.

[7] Foroutan A. Medical review of Iraqi chemical warfare: abstract. In: Foroutan A, editor. Medical review of Iraqi chemical warfare. Tehran: Baqiyatallah University of Medical Sciences; 2004. p. i–viii.

[8] Zilinskas RA. Iraq's biological weapons: the past as future? JAMA 1997;278:418–24.

[9] Eitzen EM, Takafuji ET. Historical overview of biological warfare. In: Sidell FR, Takafuji ET, Franz DR, editors. Medical aspects of chemical and biological warfare. Washington (DC): The Office of the Surgeon General at TMM publications; 1997. p. 415–23.

[10] Christopher GW, Cieslak TJ, Pavlin JA, et al. Biological warfare: a historical perspective. JAMA 1997;278:412–7.

[11] Henderson DA, Inglesby TV, Bartless JG, et al. Smallpox as a biological weapon: medical and public health management. JAMA 1999;281:2127–37.

[12] Meselson M, Guillemin J, Hugh-Jones M, et al. The Sverdlosk anthrax outbreak of 1979. Science 1994;266:1202–8.

[13] Alibek K. Biohazard. New York: Random House, Inc.; 1999.

[14] Arnon SS, Schechter R, Inglesby TV, et al. Botulinum toxin as a biological weapon: medical and public health management. JAMA 2001;285:1059–70.

[15] Hogan DE, Kellison T. Nuclear terrorism. Am J Med Sci 2002;323:341–9.

[16] Ring JP. Radiation risks and dirty bombs. Radiat Safety J 2004;86:S42–7.

[17] Yablokov A. Testimony of Dr. Alexie Yablokov. Washington (DC): United States House National Security Committee; 1997.

[18] Morita H, Yanagisawa N, Nakajima T, et al. Sarin poisonin in Matsumoto, Japan. Lancet 1995;346:290–3.

[19] Okumura T, Suzuki K, Fukuda A, et al. The Tokyo subway sarin attack: disaster management, part 2: hospital response. Acad Emerg Med 1998;5:618–24.

[20] Okumura T, Takasu N, Ishimatsu S, et al. Report on 6409 victims of the Tokyo subway sarin attack. Ann Emerg Med 1996;28:129–35.

[21] Dhara VR, Dhara R. The Union Carbide disaster in Bhopal: a review of health effects. Arch Environ Health 2002;57:391–404.

[22] Varma DR, Guest I. The Bhopal accident and methyl isocyanate toxicity. J Toxicol Environ Health 1993;40:513–29.

[23] Torok TJ, Tauxe RV, Wise RP, et al. A large comunity outbreak of Salmonellosis caused by intentional contamination of restaurant salad bars. JAMA 1997;278:389–95.

[24] Keim P, Smith KL, Keys C, et al. Molecular investigation of the Aum Shinrikyo anthrax release in Kameido, Japan. J Clin Microbiol 2001;39:4566–7.

[25] Inglesby TV, O'Toole T, Henderson DA, et al. Anthrax as a biological weapon, 2002: updated recommendations for management. JAMA 2002;287:2236–52.

[26] Burgess JL, Kovalchick DF, Harter L, et al. Hazardous materials events: evaluation of transport to health care facility and evacuation decisions. Am J Emerg Med 2001;19:99–105.

[27] Berkowitz Z, Horton DK, Kaye WE. Hazardous substances causing fatalities and/or people transported to hospitals: rural/agricultural vs. other areas. Prehosp Disast Med 2004;19: 213–20.

[28] Horton DK, Berkowitz Z, Kaye WE. Surveillance of hazardous materials events in 17 states, 1993–2001: a report from the Hazardous Substances Emergency Events Surveillance (HSEES) System. Am J Ind Med 2004;45:539–48.

[29] Richards CF, Burstein JL, Waeckerle JF, et al. Emergency physicians and biological terrorism. Ann Emerg Med 1999;34:183–90.

[30] Greenberg MI, Hendrickson RG. Report of the CIMERC/Drexel University Emergency Department Terrorism Preparedness Consensus Panel. Acad Emerg Med 2003;10:783–8.

ELSEVIER
SAUNDERS

Crit Care Clin 21 (2005) 653–672

CRITICAL
CARE
CLINICS

Decontamination

Marc Houston, DO[a], Robert G. Hendrickson, MD[b],*

[a]*Oregon Health and Science University, CDW-EM, 3181 S.W. Sam Jackson Park Road,
Portland, OR 97239, USA*
[b]*Oregon Health and Science University, Oregon Poison Control, CSB-550,
3181 S.W. Sam Jackson Park Road, Portland, OR 97239, USA*

During a terrorist-related disaster, victims may become contaminated with chemical (eg, chlorine), biologic (eg, anthrax spores), or radiologic (eg, cesium-137) agents. In these scenarios, it is imperative to separate the victims from the potential causative agent to decrease the risks to the treating health care workers and to the patients themselves. Decontamination is the reduction or removal of harmful substances from the body [1]. The primary goal of decontamination is to eliminate substances from the skin, hair, mucosal surfaces, lungs, and gastro-intestinal (GI) tract so that the agent is neither absorbed by the patient nor is transferred to the treating health care workers or rescuers. We will discuss here the indications for, and the process of, decontamination of victims of chemical, biologic, and radiologic (CBR) agents.

During a disaster or hazardous materials accident, decontamination is normally performed either by hazardous material (HAZMAT) or emergency medical service (EMS) personnel, or by the staff in the hospital emergency department [2]. Although decontamination should preferentially occur outside of the hospital environment [3], the sarin attack in Tokyo, Japan [4,5], and the SARS cases in Singapore [6] are examples of instances where critical care professionals were involved with patients who required the principles of decontamination and personal protective equipment.

Incidents involving the principles of CBR exposures such as hazardous materials spills, industrial chemical releases, and industrial exposures to radioisotopes occur commonly in the United States, and can affect critical care professionals regardless of their geographic location or perceived risk of terrorist attack.

* Corresponding author.
E-mail address: hendriro@ohsu.edu (R.G. Hendrickson).

Over 4 billion tons of chemicals are transported per year in the United States [7]. Large quantities of phosgene, cyanide, ammonia, and chlorine, are stored and transported frequently on interstate highways and rail lines [8–10]. In fact, over 32,000 acute releases of hazardous chemicals occur in the United States per year [11], with an associated 1.6 transportation-related hazardous materials incidents that result in death, injury, or evacuation each year [12]. Radiologic waste from power plants, military, and industrial uses is also transported by rail and truck throughout the United States. With this in mind, it is important for critical care professionals to thoroughly understand the principles and performance of decontamination, as well as its limitations, [13] for several reasons:

1. Critical care professionals may need to care for patients who have been decontaminated in the prehospital or emergency department setting.
2. In an overwhelming disaster, critical care professionals may need to care for patients in the emergency department or in proximity to decontamination.
3. Critical care professionals may need to ensure that the patients for whom they are caring are fully decontaminated before transfer to the critical care unit.
4. In certain rare circumstances, critical care professionals may need to care for patients in their critical care unit who are contaminated, and may require additional decontamination of the skin, lungs, or GI tract.

The information below is not sufficient or intended to provide expertise in decontamination or personal protective equipment (PPE). Decontamination is a physical exercise that requires significant, and repeated, hands-on training. In addition, it is not our intention to imply that critical care professionals should be performing primary hospital decontamination, as this would be an inappropriate use of the skills of highly trained health care workers [3]. Our aim is to describe the reasons for decontamination, as well as the process of decontamination, to facilitate a better comprehension of these procedures.

Decontamination

In the event of a hazardous materials accident or a CBR release, procedures and protocols are put into action by the local or regional HAZMAT team(s) responding to the incident. Most procedures and protocols for on-scene prehospital (EMS or HAZMAT team) decontamination are patterned after the military model consisting of zones: hot, warm, and cold [14,15]. The hot zone is the area of highest contamination or that area immediately surrounding the point of contact with the contaminant. Within the hot zone there may be a potentially dangerous amount of an agent either on surfaces or in the air. All rescuers entering this area wear the highest level of PPE (Table 1) needed for the exposure; a self-contained (Level A) splash-proof garment with supplied oxygen [12]. This level of PPE protects the rescuer from gases, aerosols, vapor, solids,

Table 1
Personal protective equipment

Level	Protects against these materials	Respiratory equipment	Skin protection	Scenario where this level is useful/necesssary
A	Gases, vapors, aerosols, oxygen-deficient areas, liquids, and solids	Self-contained breathing apparatus (SCBA) (protection from gas, vapor, or oxygen-deficient environment)	Fully encapsulated, chemical resistant suit (protection from vapor)	Entering a prehospital hot zone that is oxygen deficient or is filled with potentially toxic gas or vapor (eg, prehospital rescue from a hot zone)
B	Vapors, aerosols, oxygen-deficient areas, solids, and liquids	SCBA or positive pressure supplied-air respirator (SAR) (protection from gas, vapor or oxygen-deficient environments)	Splash-proof, chemical resistant suit (protection from splashes)	Entering a prehospital decontamination zone (warm) that is oxygen deficient, contains potentially toxic gases, or where there is a risk of splashes from potentially toxic solids or liquids
C	Most vapors and aerosols, solids, and liquids	(Powered) Air-purifying respirator (APR or PAPR) or face cartridge mask	Splash-proof chemical resistant suit (protection from splashes)	Operating in an environment where the main threat is liquid or solid or low concentration of select vapors (recommended for hospital-based decontamination)
D	None	HEPA filter protects against particulate matter	Minimal	Universal precautions appropriate for fully decontaminated patient (eg, postdecontamination care)

and liquids. Patients in the hot zone are located and taken out to the warm zone. Only basic life-saving treatments are initiated in this area such as basic airway control, hemorrhage control, and any antidotal therapy, if necessary. Patients are decontaminated in the warm zone. This area is usually placed a distance from the hot zone, if at all possible uphill and upwind. It is expected that the warm zone will have some amount of contamination, but much less than that in the hot zone. Initiation of medical treatment is still very limited in the warm zone with interventions sufficient only to stabilize the patients long enough to be effectively decontaminated and moved to the cold zone. The cold zone is designated as safe and free from contamination. It is anticipated that all patients who arrive in this area have been properly decontaminated and are available for full medical treatment. No contaminated equipment or clothing, including contamination on patient skin, should pass from the warm zone into the cold zone [14]. Criticisms of the military model include that it is too labor intensive and time consuming to be used effectively in a hospital or civilian setting.

Although many patients may be decontaminated at the scene by HAZMAT and EMS professionals as described above, the majority of patients arriving to hospitals after acute events are self-transported and have *not* been decontaminated by prehospital personnel [3,4]. Decontamination of these patients is required before entering the hospital setting [3,16]. Decontamination at a hospital differs from the prehospital/military model in several important ways.

Patients arriving to the hospital have traveled away from the exposure and therefore, away from the hot zone [16,17]. For that reason, there is no hot zone in hospital-based decontamination. In addition, patients who are exposed to agents typically begin to arrive at hospitals approximately 20 minutes or more after their exposure [3,4]. In that time, the patient has been out of the hot zone and has possibly been partially decontaminated by evaporation of the agent off the skin [18]. The quantity of contaminant that hospital personnel may encounter is therefore dramatically less than the quantity to which the victim was initially exposed [1]. Given this, the hospital decontamination procedure begins with a lower risk of secondary contamination than in the prehospital setting [17,19].

The minimum required PPE for hospital-based decontamination when dealing with an unknown hazardous substance includes a chemically resistant suit sealed with tape, double-layer protective gloves, and a power air-purifying respirator (PAPR) using combination high-efficiency particulate air/organic vapor/ acid respiratory cartridges [17,19]. Higher levels of protection may be considered necessary based upon specific community hazards [17,19].

Skin decontamination—methods and effectiveness

Decontamination of the skin is the primary intervention needed for the majority of CBR exposures [20]. Patients exposed to liquids, aerosols, or solids will likely require skin decontamination [14,20]. Exposure to gases or vapor does not require decontamination [1,20,21], as removal of the affected patient from the area is all that is required [1]. However, patients who are exposed to vapor should have their clothing removed in case the vapor has condensed on their clothing [21], and so that they do not expose the workers caring for them [1].

Unfortunately, it is generally not possible to identify an agent or the properties of an agent (eg, gas, liquid, aerosol, and so on) during an acute event in the hospital setting [22]. Given this, it is likely prudent to decontaminate all patients in the hospital setting if there is a possibility of contamination and resources are not overwhelmed. If resources and decontamination facilities are limited or overwhelmed, an alternative strategy is to allow patients to exchange their contaminated clothing for clean clothing (gown or scrubs) in a sheltered area until they can be tested or decontaminated [23].

The decontamination process begins with the removal of clothing [1,17, 23–25]. As with any evaluation of a patient, requiring removal of clothing, modesty, patient privacy, and protection from hypothermia are important [16]. Privacy screening and warm water should be used [16]. Removal of the victim's clothing may be the most important step in decontamination, as it can reduce the quantity of contaminant associated with the victim by an estimated 75 to 90% [12,26], depending on the amount of clothing the patient was wearing at the time of the exposure. Clothes are cut, rather than pulled, off as pulling can increase the area of contamination and exposure to the victim and surrounding health care providers [17]. Tugging and tearing the clothes may also produce an aerosol of the agent that may increase the exposure of the patient as well as the health care provider. In addition, cutting the clothing avoids exposing the facial mucous membranes, nose, and mouth to any agent that is on the shirt as it is removed over the head. Removal of clothing is considered to be the minimum level and most important part of decontamination for all victims of a chemical or radiologic incident [1,5].

Once the clothing is removed, it should be labeled with a patient identifier, sealed within plastic bags, and stored [16]. Sealing and storing the clothing will prevent evaporation or aerosolization of the agent in the hospital area [1]. Labeling the bags will allow the patient to potentially retrieve items such as a wallet and other identification items. In addition, labeling permits testing of the clothing for the agent as may be required for a criminal investigation [16]. Labeling may also allow for epidemiologic evaluation of the release by identifying the agent on clothing and matching that information to the location of the patient at the time of the release.

The next step in decontamination is the cleaning of the skin, which is most effectively achieved by physically removing the offending agent [20,27]. Solids can be physically removed by using a soft brush or towel, and the skin should be thoroughly washed with copious warm water and soap [16,17]. Timely flushing or flooding of the contaminated skin with copious amounts of fluid physically removes and significantly dilutes the agent [1,20,24,28]. The use of water flushes is effective even for highly volatile and potent agents. In one study, 10.6 times the lethal dose of contamination with sarin (GD) was required to kill test subjects that were rapidly flushed with water compared with those who were not decontaminated [27]. In addition, a 2-minute soap and water decontamination decreased absorption of the pesticide azodrin from 14% to 2% when performed 15 minutes after application [28].

Although several decontamination solutions have been proposed in the past, virtually all agents can be safely and effectively decontaminated by brushing off solids and flushing with copious amounts of water and soap [1,14,16,17,20,27]. There are a few substances that react violently with water and have been theorized as contraindications to water decontamination, including lithium, metallic sodium, potassium, cesium, and rubidium [1]. Nonetheless, the rapid and copious irrigation of these substances is still safer than delaying physical removal to use special decontamination methods, as the time to removal of the agent is the most important factor in decreasing exposure [27]. As stated above, knowledge of the specific agent used in an overt terrorist event may not be possible in the early stages of the event [22]. However, it is not necessary to positively identify the agent before decontamination, as physical removal with large volumes of liquid will work equally as well regardless of the chemical's characteristics [20,21].

In addition to physical removal of agents, flushing with water during dermal decontamination may produce some chemical deactivation of the agent, although this is probably not clinically relevant in the hospital setting [20]. Chemical deactivation refers to the role of the fluid in producing a chemical reaction that neutralizes the toxicity of the agent. Chemical deactivation, including hydrolysis and oxidative chlorination of chemical agents are theoretically possible and have been studied, but are likely not effective means of chemical removal because these reactions require a significant contact time [20,27]. Hydrolysis may occur with the addition of acidic or alkaline solutions, and is effective in deactivating nerve agents [20,27]. However, clinically significant hydrolysis is slow, and only occurs when solutions are used that have a pH that is not acceptable for use on skin or mucosa (ie, pH 10–11) [20,27]. Oxidative chlorination may occur with the addition of a dilute (0.5%) bleach solution. The military continues to recommend using a freshly made dilute, alkaline 0.5% hypochlorite solution for decontamination [20,27,29]. Dilute bleach has been proven effective in oxidizing mustard agent and organic phosphorous compounds [20,27]. However, oxidative chlorination requires an unacceptable amount of time to occur on the skin with most agents [20,27], and dilute bleach cannot be used in eyes or on mucosal surfaces making it an undesirable decontamination solution in the hospital setting [20,27]. Showering with soap and water is widely considered to be effective, and is the preferred method for removal of chemical agents from contaminated individuals skin and hair [15,27], due to its efficacy and ready availability in the hospital setting.

The addition of soap to decontamination has several potential, but largely unproven, advantages over using water alone. For a few specific agents, soap has been shown to enhance removal of the substance from the skin [30,31]; however, most agents have not been tested. Certain alkaline soaps (eg, "green soap") may add some degree of chemical hydrolysis to the decontamination effort. Although this likely does not occur rapidly enough to decrease the patient's exposure, soap may continue to hydrolyze in the water runoff, thus theoretically decreasing bystander and environmental exposure. More importantly than any chemical effect, soap reminds patients to physically wipe all areas of the body, including areas that are typically missed during decontamination procedures, such as groin, hair, axilla, and feet.

If the eyes have been exposed to a chemical or radiologic agent or biologic toxin, they should be decontaminated as early as is possible after the exposure. Remove contact lenses if removal can be accomplished easily and without additional trauma to the eye. Flush the eyes with water or normal saline immediately for about 20 minutes by tilting the head to the side, pulling eyelids apart with fingers, and pouring water slowly into eyes. Flushing may alternatively be performed using specially designed lenses (eg, Morgan lenses) that fit under the eyelids and allow for hands-free flushing. If a corrosive material is suspected or if pain or injury is evident, the pH of the surface of the eye should be recorded and irrigation continued until the pH is 7. Do not cover eyes with bandages.

Several alternative methods of decontamination have been studied, and may be useful in specific circumstances. Dry decontamination uses the topical application of a solid, such as activated charcoal (AC), flour, or Fuller's Earth, to bind, or adsorb, the agent. The agent and the solid are then removed physically by a brush or towel. Both flour and Fuller's Earth effectively decrease absorption of chemical agents, including the nerve agents GD (soman) and VX, as well as HD (sulfur mustard) [27,32]. Alternatively, the United States military uses a carbonaceous adsorbent and ion-exchange resins in a packet referred to as M-291 resin for local, dermal decontamination [20,27]. Dry decontamination may be an effective method of removing small amounts of a topical agent, but is likely not a viable alternative method for large-scale, full-body decontamination in the hospital setting. Dry decontamination has a theoretical role in regions where environmental exposure may be hazardous to patients (eg, freezing temperatures) or in the prehospital setting [23]. However, a more reasonable hospital-based solution in freezing temperatures may be to have patients disrobe just before entering the hospital, and to shower inside [23]. Regardless of the ambient temperature, people who have been exposed to a life-threatening amount of chemical contamination should disrobe, undergo decontamination with copious amounts of high-volume, low-pressure water, or an alternative decontamination method; this should be followed by appropriate sheltering as soon as possible [23].

Decontamination time

Despite the volume of information regarding CBR terrorism, there is no benchmark standard for duration of decontamination [17]. The majority of the information regarding decontamination and duration is available from the military. The suggested duration of decontamination in published guidelines ranges from between 3 to 5 minutes [33–36] to 15 to 30 minutes [12,27,37]. The United States Army Center of Health Promotion and Preventative Medicine advocates a tepid water rinsing from head to toe for 1 minute after contaminated clothing is removed. A more thorough decontamination including washing with soap and water should follow. The United States Army Soldier and Biologic Chemical Command's Mass Casualty Decontamination Research Team states that ideally, actual showering duration might last as long as 2 to 3 minutes per patient. The Agency for Toxic Substances and Disease Registry proposes that patients contaminated with an unidentified agent should flush exposed or irritated skin and hair with plain water for a period of 2 to 5 minutes. Chemicals that are oily or adherent should be washed with mild soap followed by a thorough rinse with water. The military recommends continuing flushing until certification that the chemical is decontaminated by use of the Chemical Agent Monitor, M-8 paper or M-9 paper [27]. The use of chemical detection paper to certify decontamination may be appropriate for a single individual patient decontamination in a military model, but may be more problematic to do operationally during a mass casualty incident depending on the hospital's resources, personnel, and access to these items [5].

Little research has been performed to determine the optimal decontamination time in a hospital setting. One retrospective review of a hospital-based decontamination protocol that included a 3-minute low-volume, low-pressure shower with detergent was used on 72 patients over a 6-year period. Ten of 31 patients who were skin-swab tested before decontamination tested positive (eight for pesticides and two for polychlorinated biphenyls). All 10 patients with an initial detectable agent had no detectable agent after the 3-minute decontamination [34]. An in vivo study of the dermal absorption of pesticides showed that a 2-minute soap and water wash decreased absorption of the pesticide azodrin from 14.7% to 2.3%, parathion from 36.3% to 7.1%, and Lindane from 9.3% to 1.8% when administered 15 minutes after application [28]. Chemical simulants of terrorist agents have been used to test the efficacy of soap and water decontamination in a hospital center. This decontamination eliminated the chemical simulants of sarin (simulant = ethyl lactate) and sulfur mustard (simulant = methyl salicylate) entirely within 3 to 6 minutes [35]. In the same study, the water-soluble chemical (ethyl lactate) was entirely removed with a 3-minute water shower without soap [35].

Studies on radioisotopes also suggest that rapid washing with water and soap is the ideal method of decontamination, but that detergents may be effective for particular isotopes. A 15-second wash with soap and water is effective in decreasing Tc^{99} on skin by 78% to 99% [30,38]; however, other isotopes, including I^{123} and Cr^{51} require longer washing (reduction of 88% after 2 minutes) [38]. For some isotopes, the addition of a detergent may expedite removal [38]. For radioisotopes that are common in medical practice (Tc^{99}, I^{131}, Ga^{57}, In^{111}), a 90-second water rinse with or without soap eliminates over 90% of the agent [31]. In most situations, it seems reasonable that a 3-to 6-minute shower with soap and water is sufficient to eliminate all the radioisotope that is possible to remove without special techniques [33]. Detecting less than two times the baseline counts per minute (cpm) or less than 100 cpm over a 10 cm^2 area with a radiation survey meter (eg, Geiger-Muller counter) following decontamination determines completion of the decontamination process after radioisotope contamination [39].

In 2004, the Occupational Safety and Health Administration (OSHA) published the most comprehensive guidelines for hospital-based decontamination [17]. In this document, OSHA suggests a 5- to 6-minute rinse for an unknown chemical; however, this recommendation is based on the opinion of experts and not on published evidence [17]. It is likely that 5 to 6 minutes of decontamination would remove the vast majority of possible agents that might be encountered in a hospital, even in critically ill patients who are likely to have more contamination than the other patients reporting to the hospital. However, there is a paucity of evidence in the medical literature concerning hospital-based decontamination, particularly for intensive care patients, so we propose a common-sense solution for postdecontamination care of critically ill patients. Patients who require critical care should be decontaminated for approximately 5 to 6 minutes with water and soap. Asymptomatic patients or patients exposed to biologic agents may require much shorter decontamination times (eg, 2 to 3 minute wash with soap and water), but for critically ill patients it is prudent to assume massive contamination [36]. Health care workers who care for critically ill patients after decontamination should don PPE that is appropriate for universal precautions to body fluids. The patient should be thoroughly examined, and if the patient has visible agent on their skin, mucosa, or hair, then the patient requires additional decontamination. If chemical skin testing is available, then evidence of agent on the skin determines the need for additional decontamination. Naturally, if any health care worker who is caring for the patient develops any symptoms, then those health care workers should don Level-C PPE and the patient would require additional decontamination. Additional alternatives are to investigate what your local disaster protocols recommend or contact the regional poison control center for further guidance [14]. Poison control centers are an important resource for critical care professionals, as they provide critical information concerning agent characteristics, toxicology, clinical effects, and medical management [3,22,40].

Risk of secondary contamination to the health care worker

During victim decontamination procedures, the hazard to health care workers is due only to secondary exposure to contaminant on the patient or vapor from the patient's skin, hair, or clothing. In general, the health risk is low for a hospital provider caring for contaminated patients [19,41]. However, there are certainly cases where the treatment of contaminated patients within a hospital has lead to not only illness in the hospital workers (secondary contamination and injury), but even hospital closures [4,19,42–47]. There are several preventable reasons why medical personnel in these cases have historically been affected, including failure to remove patient clothing, failure to perform appropriate decontamination, and failure to don appropriate PPE suitable for the level of patient contamination [17,44–47]. Secondary exposures have usually involved common hazardous materials, as well as volatile substances, such as organic phosphorous compounds (including sarin), chlorine, acids, and hydrocarbons [19,45,46]. However, even particulate matter may produce secondary contamination. In one simulation of the treatment of a single contaminated patient in a hospital decontamination facility, those performing decontamination were exposed (in their breathing space) to a volatile chemical (xylene and acetone) as well as particulate matter (iron and zinc oxide) from the patient's clothing during treatment. Although the exposure to these health care workers was fairly small, it was a reminder that exposure to chemicals or particulate matter (eg, radioisotope or biologic agents) is possible without prior decontamination [41]. In one hospital during the Tokyo sarin attacks, 23% of all health care workers in the hospital developed symptoms because patients were not required to remove clothing, were not decontaminated, and the hospital employees wore little PPE [4]. In another hospital during the same event, 13 of 15 physicians caring for victims developed symptoms, including six with cough, dyspnea, or chest tightness, and six who received atropine [44]. These physicians spent a significant amount of time caring for a small group of critically ill patients who likely had significant amounts of agent on their skin and clothing.

Particulate (biologic and radiologic) agents are decontaminated with the same approach as liquid chemical agents [1]. The majority of the difference between these exposures is the time frame in which they occur. After a single, acute release of an agent (CBR) that produces rapid onset symptoms (eg, chlorine, nerve agent, cyanide, or a dirty bomb), patients present to health care with contaminant on their clothing and skin. In addition, patients may report to health care facilities after an announced (overt) or discovered (covert) acute release of an agent that does not produce rapid symptoms [16]. However, in the case of a delayed onset agent (eg, botulinum toxin, staphylococcal enterotoxin B) or an exposure to a biologic that has a long incubation period (eg, anthrax), patients reporting to the hospital may no longer be externally contaminated, may have no risk of secondary contamination, and may not require decontamination [16]. This is particularly true for covert releases of biologic agents with long incubation periods, as they do not seek health care for several days after exposure, and have likely bathed and changed clothing several times since the exposure.

Internal decontamination—methods and effectiveness

Internal decontamination is defined as removal of contaminants from the pulmonary and GI systems. The primary purpose of internal decontamination is to either decrease absorption of the substance or to decrease mucosal exposure to the agent (eg, radioisotopes). Internal decontamination may be necessary in cases where the patient has been exposed to an agent via the pulmonary system, where the agent is causing continued damage, and is not capable of rapidly diffusing out of the pulmonary system. The prime example of this scenario is the rare instance of the inhalation of a radioisotope. Internal decontamination may also be necessary when the GI tract is exposed to a chemical, biologic, or radiologic agent via ingestion. This scenario may occur with the contamination of food or water supplies or a covert aerial exposure to an agent.

Gastrointestinal decontamination

GI decontamination is defined as the removal of potentially harmful substances from within the GI tract to decrease absorption or to increase excretion. GI decontamination in terrorist events may be necessary when exposure to the CBR agent occurs via ingestion. Alternatively, some agents, particularly radioisotopes, may be ingested after exposure of the mucosa and pulmonary tree, with resulting coughing and swallowing. GI decontamination may be performed by gastric lavage to empty the stomach, by using AC to adsorb agents, via whole bowel irrigation to push the agent through the GI tract before absorption, or via binding agents to chelate radioisotopes within the GI tract.

Gastric lavage is a method of stomach emptying that is used with the intent of decreasing passage of substances to the intestines and avoiding absorption. Gastric lavage is rarely used in acute overdoses of medication, and is typically performed using a 30 French orogastric tube. In experimental animal studies, lavage may decrease absorption by 26% to 37% [48–51]; however, human studies have not demonstrated a consistent effect on patient outcome [52–54]. Due to significant evidence of morbidity including aspiration, laryngospasm, and esophageal perforation [55], lavage should not be used unless the GI toxin is life threatening and the procedure can be completed within 1 hour of ingestion [55]. Given these limitations, it is unlikely for lavage to be effective in critical care patients.

AC is a fine black powder that is commonly used to adsorb ingested substances. AC is carbonaceous material that is pyrolyzed, then oxidized with carbon dioxide, steam, and heat to create a porous surface with massive surface area [56]. AC is capable of binding to multiple substances via hydrogen bonding, dipole, ion–ion, and van der Waals' forces [57]. AC has been shown to decrease the absorption of a variety of substances [56]. Although little specific testing has been performed, there is evidence that AC is capable of adsorption to many of the agents and radioisotopes that are likely to contaminate the GI tract [58–61] (Table 2); however, poor binding has been described with ricin [62] and Cesium-137 [63]. AC has been shown to decrease absorption of several pharmaceutical agents by 89% if given within 30 minutes and 37% if given within 1 hour of ingestion [56]. AC binds poorly to a select handful of substances including substances that are small, polar, water soluble molecules, or dissociated salts [57], such as iron, lithium, and alcohols [57].

AC is safe when used as described [64–67]. The main side effect is aspiration [68,69], and this is generally seen in patients with alterations of mental status

Table 2
Affinity of activated charcoal adsorption of selected potential GI terrorist agents

Agent	Binding capacity to activated charcoal
Cyanide	Poor in vitro binding, but decreased mortality in animal studies [80]
Aflatoxin	In vitro adsorption (1 mg aflatoxin to 100 mg AC) [58], only effective in animal models with large AC doses [81]
Ricin	Poor binding due to the size of the molecule (66 kDa) [82]
Staphylococcal Enterotoxin B	Likely to be poor due to the size of the molecule (28.5 kDa) [82]
T-2 tricothecene mycotoxin	Good in vitro adsorption (0.48 mg T-2 to 1 mg AC) [66] and decreased mortality in mice [61]
Botulinum toxin	Likely to be poor due to the size of the molecule (150 kDa) [82]
Radioisotopes with GI absorption (% of dose absorbed)	
Iodine-131 (100% GI absorption)	Evidence for in vitro, nonmedical I-131 binding to AC, but no studies on medical uses [59]
Cobalt-60 (5% GI absorption)	Evidence for in vitro, nonmedical Co-60 binding to AC, but no studies on medical uses [60]
Cesium-137 (100% GI absorption)	None (0 mg Ce-137 to 1000 mg AC) [63]

Abbreviation: GI, gastrointestinal.

and depression of the gag reflex [69]. Rarely, bezoar formation, or intestinal obstruction has occurred after multiple doses of AC, but has never been reported with a single dose [56]. AC is contraindicated in patients who do not have a protected airway [56] (either self-protected or protected by a cuffed endotracheal tube) or in patients who are at high risk of seizures or loss of consciousness (due to aspiration risks) or with intractable vomiting. AC is not contraindicated when GI caustic injury is present, although it should be used cautiously as it may obscure endoscopic visualization and may induce vomiting. AC may be used in patients with caustic injury if the agent is a systemic toxin and the risks of absorption of the agent outweigh the risks of vomiting and obscured endoscopy [56]. AC is typically administered as a water-based slurry in a dose of 50 g for adults, 1 g/kg body weight for children, either by mouth or via nasogastric tube [56]. This dose may be repeated every 4 hours if necessary, such as if there is evidence of a retained GI agent. Administration of AC is significantly more effective when given early after ingestion [56], and has little efficacy more than 3 hours after ingestion unless passage through the GI tract or gastric emptying is delayed. However, in the case where there is evidence of a toxin that remains in the GI tract (eg, detection of a GI radioisotope) with no contraindications, AC may be given long after ingestion.

GI decontamination may also be performed with whole-bowel irrigation (WBI). WBI entails the enteral administration of polyethylene glycol electrolyte solution (PEG-ES) in an effort to flush the toxin through the GI tract before its absorption [70]. WBI decreases the absorption of several medications by up to

73% in volunteer studies [70–72]. In a terrorist event, WBI may be indicated specifically if radioisotope is evident in the patient's GI tract. PEG-ES solution is typically administered via nasogastric tube [73] at a rate of 1.5 to 2 L/h (500 mL/h between 9 months to 6 years; 1 L/h between 6 and 12 years), and is continued until the toxin is cleared, or until the rectal effluent is clear [73]. PEG-ES solution is not absorbed and does not induce electrolyte or fluid shifts, and may be continued for extended periods of time with no ill effects. WBI is contraindicated if the patient's airway is not protected (due to aspiration risk), or has intractable vomiting, or if there is evidence of bowel perforation, obstruction, or ileus [73].

After exposure to certain radioisotopes, it may be beneficial to administer medications or chelators orally to bind to the radioisotope within the GI tract to avoid absorption. Examples of this include Prussian Blue (ferrihexacyano-ferrate[II]) for cesium-137 [74], thallium or rubidium [39], magnesium sulfate for radium-226 [75], aluminum hydroxide for phosphorous-32 [75], and Aluminum phosphate for strontium-90 exposure [75].

Pulmonary decontamination

Pulmonary decontamination may be necessary in cases where a radioisotope has been inhaled and remains present in the pulmonary tree [39]. This decontamination entails performing broncho-alveolar lavage (BAL) in the typical fashion in an attempt to remove radioisotope that is juxtaposed to the pulmonary mucosa. The usefulness of this procedure is limited to radioisotopes that are insoluble and will not clear from the pulmonary tree [74]. Health care workers who are performing the BAL should wear splash-proof PPE including gloves, cap, facemask, and booties. This PPE should be reviewed with the hospital Radiation Safety Officer before use. The lavage fluid should also be isolated and handled by the hospital Radiation Safety Officer, who can arrange for appropriate identification and disposal.

Wound decontamination

Decontamination of wounds may be necessary if wounds are contaminated with either radioisotope or chemicals. Wound contamination may be particularly difficult to resolve, and may be present even after thorough external skin decontamination. Wound decontamination entails both cleansing the wound with water and possible surgical removal of contaminant.

The initial steps in wound decontamination involve copious flushing of the wound with soap and water as well as thorough exploration of the wound. All members of the decontamination team should wear appropriate PPE as discussed above for skin decontamination. If any question exists, assume Level-C PPE that includes complete splash protection as well as a PAPR. In the case of a chemical, the goal is to eliminate the risk to the treating health care workers to be exposed to the chemical and to decrease the exposure of the patient. Typically, copious water irrigation directly into the wound with soap is sufficient for chemical removal. In the case of a foreign body, the wound should be thoroughly flushed and the foreign body should be removed with instruments (not with the hands) [27]. The main risk to the health care worker during wound decontamination is the risk of exposure to a liquid or foreign body within the wound [27]. The risk from evaporation ("off-gassing") from chemically contaminated fragments and cloth in wounds is not significant [20], and there is no risk of vapor release from contaminated wounds that do not contain foreign bodies [20,27].

In the case of radioisotope contamination, copious water irrigation directly into the wound is often sufficient to reduce the radioisotope load in the wound. Care must be taken to avoid placing a hand in or near the wound [20]. Again, any manipulation of the wound should be performed using an instrument [75]. After irrigation, the radiation safety officer or other personnel familiar with the use of a radiation survey meter, should evaluate the wound for additional radioisotope. If no radioisotope is identified, the wound should be dressed. If additional radioisotope is detected, the wound may be repeatedly irrigated. If radioisotope still remains, the presence of a radioisotope-containing foreign body should be considered. If visible, this foreign body should be removed with instruments, not with the fingers, and properly disposed of by the radiation safety officer. Definitive removal may require surgical intervention.

Radiation exposure decontamination

The medical management of patients exposed to radiation will not be covered here. We will discuss the management specific to decontamination of the patient exposed to radioisotope particles. It should be noted that patients who have an external exposure to radiation (eg, an X-ray or simple radiologic device) and not exposure to particulate matter do not require external decontamination. Patients exposed to particulate radioisotope, for example from a "dirty bomb," may require decontamination. As the particulate radioisotope on the skin is not likely to cause significant damage if removed in a reasonable time frame, decontamination is largely geared toward avoiding ingestion or inhalation of the particles. Decontamination of the radiation victim can be thought of as removing particulate matter (eg, dirt) from a patient and is similar to that for exposure to a chemical, with a few exceptions.

Critically ill patients exposed to particulate radioisotope require initial removal of clothing [33,74,76]. Patients should then be surveyed to determine if they are contaminated with radioisotope. If contamination is present, or if time does not allow a thorough survey, the patient should be thoroughly washed with soap and water. Health care workers directly involved in patient decontamination should wear PPE to protect themselves from particulates and aerosols (eg, Level C PPE with splash-proof outer garments and a PAPR) [77]. Decontaminators should ensure that the splash-proof outer garments are taped together so that particulate matter cannot settle within boots, gloves, and against skin. Privacy screening and warm water should be employed [16]. Clothing should be cut and rolled away from the face of the patient to avoid exposing the mouth and eyes to radioisotope with subsequent ingestion. Clothing and belongings should be stored as with chemical decontamination, in labeled bags that are stored away from the decontamination area. Ideally, any open wounds should be covered before decontamination, although this is often not possible [27]. The patients should wash their hair in a position that does not allow the contaminated water to run down the face. Having the ambulatory patient lean forward with their head down during the hair rinse is generally effective. After the removal of clothing and rinse, the patient should be allowed to dry and should be surveyed with a radiation survey meter to ensure that radioisotope is removed [76]. It is not necessary to completely eliminate all radioisotope from the skin. All visible radioisotope should be removed, and the patient should continue decontamination until the radiation measurement using the survey meter are below a threshold level. The appropriate threshold level should be set by the local radiation safety officer, but is generally accepted as two times over the baseline reading (baseline is the reading taken in the area, but away from exposed patients) [78] or greater than 100 cpm over a 10^2 cm area of skin [39].

Victims of explosive radiation dispersal devices ("dirty bombs"), may have embedded shrapnel that contains radioisotope. In this scenario, the wound must be thoroughly explored and irrigated as described above. Despite significant decontamination, patients may retain radioisotope within wounds. This may or may not require surgical excision, depending on the amount and type of radioisotope. It is possible that the patient may require care in a critical care unit while still retaining radioisotope in a wound. It is not possible for staff to be exposed to significant amounts of radiation from a contaminated wound. Any risk to staff is from the contamination of the staff's skin with particulate matter from the wound. This risk can be eliminated if universal precautions are kept [27].

Patients who are exposed to radioisotope via the lungs (eg, as an aerosol or airborne exposure) or GI tract (eg, as a food/water contaminant, or airborne exposure with swallowing of radioisotope) may require pulmonary or GI decontamination as described above.

The major difference between the decontamination of patients exposed to radioisotope particles and those exposed to chemical or biologic agents is that patients who are exposed to an explosive radiologic dispersion device ("dirty bomb") may require medical care before decontamination. Because the risk to health care workers from exposure to a radioisotope-contaminated patient is very low, patients may require medical treatment of traumatic conditions before having any decontamination. Once again, removal of the clothing, which is inherent in trauma care, likely removes most of the particulate matter. Hospital staff attending to these potentially contaminated patients need only wear splash-proof garments (gown, gloves, hat, booties) with a facemask and eye-shield to protect themselves from ingestion or inhalation of particles or prolonged exposure of the agent to their skin. These patients may be resuscitated and then decontaminated at a later time. Unlike chemical decontamination, radiologic decontamination is not an emergency.

Summary

As the name implies, terrorists are interested in causing terror, or widespread fear and panic. Although terrorists may kill to forward their aims, their choice of agent may be more directed toward those that cause panic and terror rather than agents that kill rapidly. Large numbers of victims may only serve to provoke those they wish to terrorize. The events of September 11, 2001, and the Tokyo Sarin Subway attack opened many eyes to the extremes that terrorists will go to force their agenda.

The ability to decontaminate victims completely may be impossible given the resources available when presented with several thousand potentially exposed patients. Critical care physicians will ultimately take care of the sickest of these patients, specifically those who were the most contaminated. The truly contaminated patient may require further pulmonary, GI, or wound decontamination if they are admitted to the intensive care unit. A concrete understanding of decontamination procedures and protocols is crucial. An understanding of decontamination will steer your treatment of the contaminated patient, but also will help you to protect your staff from becoming secondarily contaminated.

Critical care clinicians should be integrated in disaster preparation and planning for their hospital and community. Decontamination is one of the foundations of disaster preparation and planning. Intensivists are aptly trained for these unique patients not only in their ability to care for them, but their multidisciplinary approach enables them to lessen early preventable mortality and foresee pitfalls in the care of CBR patients [13,79].

References

[1] Levitin HW, Siegelson HJ, Dickinson S, et al. Decontamination of mass casualties—re-evaluating existing dogma. Prehosp Disast Med 2003;18:200–7.
[2] Waeckerle J, Seamans S, Whiteside M, et al. Task force of health care and emergency services professionals on preparedness for nuclear, biological, and chemical incidents. Ann Emerg Med 2001;37:587–601.
[3] Greenberg MI, Hendrickson RG. Report of the CIMERC/Drexel University Emergency Department Terrorism Preparedness Consensus Panel. Acad Emerg Med 2003;10:783–8.
[4] Okumura T, Suzuki K, Fukuda A, et al. The Tokyo subway sarin attack: disaster management, part 2: hospital response. Acad Emerg Med 1998;5:618–24.

[5] Okumura T, Takasu N, Ishimatsu S, et al. Report on 640 victims of the Tokyo subway sarin attack. Ann Emerg Med 1996;28:129–35.

[6] Tham K. An emergency department response to severe acute respiratory syndrome: a prototype response to bioterrorism. Ann Emerg Med 2003;43:1–9.

[7] Levitin H, Siegelson H. Hazardous materials: disaster medical planning and response. Emerg Med Clin N Am 1996;14:327–48.

[8] Leffingwill S. Public health aspects of chemical warfare agents. In: Somani S, editor. Chemical warfare agents. San Diego (CA): Academic Press; 2002. p. 323–39.

[9] Bronstein A, Currance P. Emergency care for hazardous materials exposure. 2nd edition. St. Louis (MO): Mosby-Year Book; 1994.

[10] Sidell FR. Management of chemical warfare agent casualties: a handbook for emergency medical services. Bel Air (MD): H.B. Publishing; 1995.

[11] Berkowitz Z, Horton DK, Kaye WE. Hazardous substances releases causing fatalities and/or people transported to hospitals: rural/agricultural vs. other areas. Prehosp Disast Med 2004; 19:213–20.

[12] Cox R. Decontamination and management of hazardous materials exposure victims in the emergency department. Ann Emerg Med 1994;23:761–70.

[13] Johannigman J. Disaster preparedness: it's all about me. Crit Care Med 2005;33:S22–8.

[14] Brennan R, Waeckerle J, Sharp T, et al. Chemical warfare agents: emergency medical and emergency public health issues. Ann Emerg Med 1999;34:191–204.

[15] Sidell F, Patrick W, Dashiell T, et al. In: Sidell F, editors. Jane's chem-bio handbook. 2nd edition. Alexandria (VA): Jane's Information Group; 2002.

[16] Macintyre A, Christopher G, Eitzen E, et al. Weapons of mass destruction events with contaminated casualties. JAMA 1999;283:242–9.

[17] Occupational Safety and Health Administration (OSHA). Best practices for hospital-based first receivers of victims from mass casualty incidents involving the release of hazardous substances. Washington DC: Occupational Safety and Health Administration (OSHA); 2004. p. 1–32.

[18] Georgopoulos P, Fedele P, Shade P, et al. Hospital response to chemical terrorism: personal protective equipment training, and operations. Am J Ind Med 2004;46:432–45.

[19] Hick JL, Hanfling D, Burnstein JL, et al. Protective equipment for healthcare facitlity decontamination personnel: regulations, risks, and recommendations. Ann Emerg Med 2003;42: 370–80.

[20] Hurst CG. Decontamination. In: Sidell FR, Takafuji ET, Franz DR, editors. Medical aspects of chemical and biological warfare. Washington (DC): The Office of the Surgeon General at TMM Publishers; 1997. p. 351–9.

[21] Kirk MA, Cisek J, Rose SR. Emergency department response to hazardous materials incidents. Emerg Med Clin N Am 1994;12:451–61.

[22] Kales S, Christiani D. Acute chemical emergencies. N Engl J Med 2004;350:800–8.

[23] Guidelines for cold weather mass decontaminaiton during a terrorist chemical agent incident. Aberdeen (MD): US Army Soldier and Biological Chemical Comand (SBCCOM); 2002.

[24] Patient decontamination and mass triage. Research and development to improve civilian medical response. Washington (DC): Institute of Medicine, National Research Council. Chemical and Biological Terrorism; 1999. p. 97–109.

[25] Managing hazardous material incidents: Volume II—hospital emergency departments: a planning guide for the management of contaminated patients. Part III: patient management. Atlanta (GA): Agency for Toxic Substances and Disease Registry; 2005.

[26] Vogt B, Sorrensen J. How clean is safe? Improving the effectiveness of decontamination of structures and people following chemical and biological incidents—final report. Washington (DC): US Department of Energy; 2002.

[27] Decontamination. Medical management of chemical casualties handook. 3rd edition. Aberdeen Proving Ground (MD): Chemical Casualty Care Division, US Army Medical Research Institute of Chemical Defense (USAMRICD); 2000. p. 175–93.

[28] Wester R, Maibach H. In vivo percutaneous absorption and decontamination of pesticides in humans. J Toxicol Environ Health 1985;16:25–37.

[29] Cancio L. Chemical casualty decontamination by medical platoons in the 82nd Airborne Division. Mil Med 1993;158:1–5.

[30] Nishiyama H, VanTuinen R, Lukes S, et al. Survey of 99Tc contamination of laboratory personnel: hand decontamination. Radiology 1980;137:549–51.

[31] Moore P, Mettler F. Skin decontamination of commonly used medical radionuclides. J Nucl Med 1980;21:475–6.

[32] Chilcott R, Jenner J, Hotchkis S, et al. In vitro skin absorption and decontamination of sulphur mustard: comparison of human and pig-ear skin. J Appl Toxicol 2001;21:279–83.

[33] Leonard RB, Ricks RC. Emergency department radiation accident protocol. Ann Emerg Med 1980;9:462–70.

[34] Lavoie F, Coomes T, Cisek J, et al. Emergency department external decontamination for hazardous chemical exposure. Vet Hum Toxicol 1992;34:61–4.

[35] Torngren S, Persson S, Ljungquist A, et al. Personal decontamination after exposure to simulated liquid phase contaminants: functional assessment of a new unit. J Toxicol Clin Toxicol 1998; 36:567–73.

[36] Keim M, Kaufmann A. Principles for emergency response to bioterrorism. Ann Emerg Med 1999;34:177–82.

[37] Burgess JL, Kirk M, Borron SW, et al. Emergency department hazardous materials protocol for contaminated patients. Ann Emerg Med 1999;34:205–12.

[38] Merrick M, Simpson J, Liddell S. Skin decontamination—a comparison of four methods. Br J Radiol 1982;55:317–8.

[39] Force ACoRDPT. Disaster preparedness for radiology professionals: a primer for radiologists, radiation oncologists, and medical physicists. Reston (VA): American College of Radiology; 2002. p. 9–31.

[40] Hendrickson R. Terrorist chemical releases: assessment of medical risk and implications for emergency preparedness. Hum Ecol Risk Assessment 2005;11(3):1–13.

[41] Schultz M, Cisek J, Wabeke R. Simulated exposure of hospital emergency personnel to solvent vapors and respirable dust during decontaminatino of chemically exposed patients. Ann Emerg Med 1995;26:324–9.

[42] Burgess J. Hospital evacuations due to hazardous materials incidents. Am J Emerg Med 1999;17: 50–2.

[43] Nosocomial poisoning associated with emergency department treatment of organophosphate toxicity—Georgia 2000. MMWR 2001;49:1156–8.

[44] Nozaki H, Hori S, Shinozawa Y, et al. Secondary exposure of medical staff to sarin vapor in the emergency room. Intensive Care Med 1995;21:1032–5.

[45] Horton DK, Berkowitz Z, Kaye WE. Secondary contamination of ED personnel from hazardous materials events, 1995–2001. Am J Emerg Med 2003;21:199–204.

[46] Okudera H, Morita H, Iwashita T, et al. Unexpected nerve gas exposure in the city of Matsumoto: report of rescue activity in the first sarin gas terrorism. Am J Emerg Med 1997;15:527–8.

[47] Nocera A, Levitin H, Hilton J. Dangerous bodies: a case of fatal aluminum phosphide poisoning. Med J Aust 2000;173:133–5.

[48] Arnold F, Hodges J, Barta R. Evaluation of the efficacy of lavage and induced emesis in treatement. Pediatrics 1959;23:286–301.

[49] Abdallah A, Tye A. A comparison of the efficacy of emetic drugs and stomach lavage. Am J Dis Child 1967;113:571–5.

[50] Corby D, Lisciandro R, Lehman R, et al. The efficiency of methods used to evacuate the stomach after acute ingestions. Pediatrics 1967;40:871–4.

[51] Burton B, Bayer M, Barron L, et al. Comparison of activated charcoal and gastric lavage in the prevention of aspirin absorption. J Emerg Med 1984;1:411–6.

[52] Allan B. The role of gastric lavage in the treatment of patients suffering from barbiturate overdose. Med J Aust 1961;2:513–4.

[53] Comstock E, Faulkner T, Boisaubin E, et al. Studies on the efficacy of gastric lavage as practiced in a large metropolitan hospital. Clin Toxicol 1981;18:581–97.

[54] Matthew H, Mackintosh T, Tompsett S, et al. Gastric aspiration and lavage in acute poisoning. BMJ 1966;1:1333–7.

[55] Position Statement. Gastric lavage. Clin Toxicol 1997;35:711–9.

[56] Position Paper. Single-dose activated charcoal. Clin Toxicol 2005;43:61–87.

[57] Howland MA. Activated charcoal. In: Goldfrank L, Flomenbaum NE, Lewin NA, Howland MA, Hoffman RS, Nelson LS, editors. Goldfrank's toxicologic emergencies. 7th edition. New York: McGraw-Hill; 2002. p. 469–74.

[58] Decker WJ, Corby DG. Activated charcoal adsorbs aflatoxin B1. Vet Hum Toxicol 1980;22: 388–9.

[59] Langhorst S, Morris J, Miller W. Investigation of charcoal filters used in monitoring airborne radioactive I. Health Phys 1985;48:344–7.

[60] Standford N, Mellor R. Detection of 60Co in charcoal cartridges used for airborne radioiodine collection. Health Phys 1985;49:982–5.

[61] Fricke R, Jorge J. Assessment of efficacy of activated charcoal for treatment of acute T-2 toxin poisoning. J Toxicol Clin Toxicol 1990;28:421–31.

[62] Ricin. In: Kortepeter M, editor. USAMRIID's medical management of biological casualties handbook. Frederick (MD): United States Army Medical Research Institute of Infectious Diseases; 2001.

[63] Verzijl J, Joore J, van Dijk A, et al. In vitro binding characteristics for Cesium of two qualities of prussian blue, activated charcoal and resonium-A. Clin Toxicol 1992;30:215–22.

[64] Merigian K, Woodward M, Hedges J, et al. Prospective evaluation of gastric emptying in the self-poisoned patient. Am J Emerg Med 1990;8:479–83.

[65] Kulig K, Bar-Or D, Cantrill S, et al. Management of acutely poisoned patients without gastric emptying. Ann Emerg Med 1985;14:562–7.

[66] Comstock E, Boisaubin E, Comstock B, et al. Assessment of the efficacy of activated charcoal following gastric lavage in acute drug emergencies. Clin Toxicol 1982;19:149–65.

[67] Hulten B, Adams R, Askenasi R, et al. Activated charcoal in tricyclic antidepressant poisoning. Hum Toxicol 1988;7:307–10.

[68] Menzies D, Busuttil A, Prescott L. Fatal pulmonary aspiration of oral activated charcoal. BMJ 1988;297:459–60.

[69] Pond S, Lewis-Driver D, Williams G, et al. Gastric emptying in acute overdose: a prospective randomised controlled trial. Med J Aust 1995;163:345–9.

[70] Tenenbein M. Whole bowel irrigation as a gastrointestinal decontamination procedure after acute poisoning. Med Toxicol 1988;3:77–84.

[71] Kirshenbaum L, Mathews S, Sitar D, et al. Whole-bowel irrigation versus activated charcoal in sorbitol for the ingestion of modified-release pharmaceuticals. Clin Pharmacol Ther 1989; 46:264–71.

[72] Smith S, Ling L, Halstenson C. Whole-bowel irrigation as a treatment for acute lithium overdose. Ann Emerg Med 1991;20:536–9.

[73] Position Statement. Whole bowel irrigation. Clin Toxicol 1997;35:753–62.

[74] Radiation dispersal device and industrial contamination situations. Medical management of radiological casualties. 1st edition. Bethesda (MD): Military Medical Operations Office, Armed Forces Radiobiology Research Institute; 1999. p. 34–58.

[75] Medical management of radiological casualties. 1st edition. Bethesda (MD): Military Medical Operations Office, Armed Forces Radiobiology Research Institute; 1999.

[76] Jarrett D. Medical aspects of ionizing radiation weapons. Mil Med 2001;166:6–8.

[77] Schliepman R, Gerbaudo V, Castronovo F. Radiation disaster response: preparation and simulation experience at an academic medical center. J Nucl Med Technol 2004;32:22–7.

[78] Timins J, Lipoti J. Radiological terrorism. N J Med 2003;100:14–21.

[79] Roccaforte J, Cushman J. Disaster preparation and management for the intensive care unit. Curr Opin Crit Care 2002;8:607–15.

[80] Lambert R, Kindler B, Schaeffer D. The efficacy of superactivated charcoal in treating rats exposed to a lethal oral dose of potassium cyanide. Ann Emerg Med 1988;17:595–8.

[81] Huwig A, Freimund S, Kappeli O, et al. Mycotoxin detoxication of animal feed by different adsorbents. Toxicol Lett 2001;122:179–88.

[82] Biological toxins. In: Kortepeter M, Christopher G, Cieslak T, et al, editors. USAMRIID's medical management of biological casualties handbook. 4th edition. Fort Detrick (MD): Operational Medicine Division, US Army Medical Research Institute of Infectious Diseases (USAMRIID); 2001.

ELSEVIER
SAUNDERS

CRITICAL
CARE
CLINICS

Crit Care Clin 21 (2005) 673–689

Organic Phosphorus Compounds—Nerve Agents

Claudia L. Barthold, MD*, Joshua G. Schier, MD

*Georgia Poison Center, Hughes Spalding Children's Hospital, Grady Health System,
80 Jesse Hill Jr. Drive SE, Atlanta, GA 30303-3801, USA*

The twentieth century has seen the development and refinement of chemical weapons and their use in both the battlefield and in terrorist attacks. Most countries in possession of these agents have agreed to never use them, but stockpiles still exist [1]. The organic phosphorus compounds (OPCs) are a general classification of agents that includes not only the military grade nerve agents (such as sarin), but also the more common "garden variety" organic phosphorus pesticides (OPPs) such as parathion. Although these compounds are often referred to as *organophosphates*, not all possess the side chains that the term organophosphate implies [2]. As such, the broader term organic phosphorus compound is used. The military grade nerve agents (sarin, tabun, soman, VX) represent a class of chemical agents that have already been used in warfare and represent a formidable terrorist threat. However, any of the OPCs may cause severe morbidity and mortality, and could be used as a terrorist weapon.

Past use as a weapon

The synthesis of the first potentially lethal OPC, tetraethyl pyrophosphate, occurred in 1854 [2]. In the 1930s, the highly toxic OPCs, tabun, sarin, and

---

Although the terms "organophosphate" and "organophosphorus" are used widely to refer to pesticides and nerve agents, the term "organic phosphorus compound" is technically correct and will be used in this article because several chemicals in this class do not contain a phosphate molecule. For example, parathion has a thioester group attached to a phosphorus molecule and is technically not a phosphate.

* Corresponding author.
E-mail address: cbarthold@georgiapoisoncenter.org (C.L. Barthold).

doi:10.1016/j.ccc.2005.05.010   *criticalcare.theclinics.com*

soman were developed during pesticide research by the Germans. The compounds were given the names GA, GB, and GD, respectively, with the letter G standing for "German." VX (V for venomous) was discovered by the British and produced by the Americans after World War II (WWII) [3].

The first recognized use of an OPC in battle was the wartime release of nerve agents by the Iraqis during the 1980s [3]. In Japan, the Aum Shinrikyo cult was responsible for two terrorist releases of sarin during the 1990s. Seven people died, and over 200 sought medical care in 1994 after a release in the community of Matsumoto [4]. In 1995, members of the same cult intentionally placed and then punctured several containers filled with sarin in the Tokyo subway system [5]. Over 5000 people sought medical care and 12 deaths were attributed to that release. No military or terrorist releases of OPPs are reported to date, although there are several reports of human illness resulting from intentional and unintentional exposure to these agents [6–8].

Mechanism of toxicity

Proposed use as a weapon

The physical properties of the different OPCs influence how each can be used as a weapon. For instance, sarin was carried onto the trains in Tokyo as a liquid, but once released it volatilized and caused toxicity as a vapor [5,9]. VX is the least volatile, but most potent nerve agent [10]. With a half-life of up to 6 days in soil, it can contaminate an area like a battlefield for a more prolonged period of time compared with other agents [10]. Nerve agents could be remotely delivered to target locations by bomb or rocket, and exert toxicity as a vapor or aerosol [3]. Nerve agents are heavier than air; therefore, those hiding in trenches or basements after a release could be more severely affected than those on higher ground [10].

Mass poisoning events with OPPs have occurred [8,11]. Covert terrorist attacks could employ any of the OPCs to contaminate food or water supplies [12]. A variety of the OPPs are still sold commercially in the United States as well as abroad in solid, liquid, or aerosol form [13].

Method of exposure

Toxicity from exposure to the OPCs may occur through inhalation, ingestion, transdermal absorption, ocular absorption, or intravascular injection [14–18]. Minimal dermal or ocular exposures to nerve agents may produce isolated local effects; however, systemic absorption may occur in higher doses [10,14,16,18]. Environmental conditions such as ambient temperature at the time of exposure, as well as type of clothing worn by the individual, can affect an agent's volatility and rates of dermal absorption [14].

Biochemical, cellular, and systemic effects

The mechanism of action of all OPCs, including the military grade nerve agents (nerve agents) is functional inhibition of the enzyme acetylcholinesterase (AChE). In normal cholinergic transmission, the neurotransmitter, acetylcholine (ACh), is released into the synapse in response to an action potential reaching the terminal end of a cholinergic neuron. Acetylcholine is used in the pre- and postganglionic parasympathetic and sympathetic (sweat glands) nervous system, the central nervous system (CNS), and skeletal muscle motor endplates (Fig. 1) [19]. These pathways make up the cholinergic nervous system, which can be further subdivided into muscarinic and nicotinic systems, based on type of ACh receptor employed. Muscarinic target sites include glands, pulmonary, and gastrointestinal muscles, CNS (brain), and the vagus nerve. Nicotinic sites include the autonomic ganglia of the autonomic nervous system, skeletal muscles, and the spinal cord. Normally, ACh is released from the presynaptic terminal, which allows binding to cholinergic receptors on either postsynaptic neurons or target organs. It then disassociates from the receptor and undergoes rapid enzymatic hydrolysis by AChE forming acetate and choline [19,20]. Inactivation of AChE by an OPC results in greatly increased intrasynaptic ACh concen-

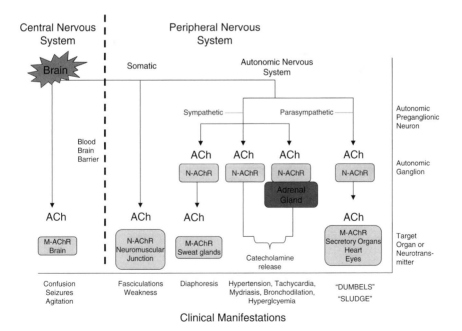

Fig. 1. Schematic depiction of human nervous system divided into its major components along with location and type of cholinergic receptor and expected clinical effects resulting from overstimulation of those receptors.

trations, resulting in overstimulation of postsynaptic neurons and target effector organs [19].

The OPCs inhibit AChE function by initially forming a reversible enzyme–inhibitor complex [21]. This complex can degrade spontaneously allowing the enzyme to be reactivated or can undergo a process known as aging [22]. Aging is a time-dependent dealkylation reaction that results in irreversible enzyme inactivation [20–24]. If administered before aging, a class of drugs known as oximes can reactivate bound AChE by removing the OPC from the OPC–AChE complex [20].

The aging rate is variable, and can be measured in minutes for soman, in hours for sarin and tabun, and in hours to days for VX. Once aging has occurred, oximes are unable to restore AChE activity and synthesis of new AChE is required to restore function [2,15,23,24]. The carbamate pesticides have a similar mechanism of action to the OPCs. They, however, do not undergo the aging process [24]. The carbamate–AChE bond is reversible, allowing for spontaneous reactivation of the enzyme after a variable agent-dependent time period.

Systemic effects

OPCs are nonspecific inhibitors of carboxylic ester hydrolases including AChE (found in nervous tissue, skeletal muscle, and on erythrocyte membranes), butyrylcholinesterase (also known as plasma or pseudocholinesterase), chymotrypsin, and other proteases [2,15,19]. The roles of each of these enzymes and their relationship to OPCs are not completely understood. In the CNS, neurotransmitters other than ACh, such as gamma-amino-butyric acid, and receptors, such as N-methyl-D-aspartate, may also be involved in the toxic effects seen after exposure to an OPC [21,25–27]. There is some evidence that muscarinic receptors on the heart are bound by nerve agents directly, but the significance is not well understood [28].

Clinical presentation

Symptoms and sequence of symptoms

The clinical presentation of ill patients is variable depending on exposure characteristics such as agent, route of exposure, dose, and receptor affinity. Signs and symptoms resulting from overstimulation of muscarinic receptors is remembered by the mneumonic DUMBELS: diaphoresis and diarrhea, urination, miosis, bradycardia, bronchorrhea, bronchospasm, emesis, lacrimation, and salivation and secretion [2,16,29,30]. Nicotinic signs and symptoms include mydriasis, muscle fasciculations, generalized muscle cramps, pallor, flaccid paralysis, hypertension, and tachycardia [2,16,29,30]. CNS effects are both neurologic and behavioral, and include giddiness, insomnia, tension, anxiety, emotional liability, central respiratory depression, convulsions, coma, and ataxia [16,21,30–32].

The most likely routes of exposure in a terrorist attack, especially for the nerve agents, would probably be either inhalational or dermal. Generally, similar signs and symptoms should occur regardless of the route of exposure, after systemic absorption. Minimal vapor exposure may only yield local eye irritation, miosis, or rhinorrhea [9,30]. As the exposure intensity from vapor increases, upper airway and then lower airway symptoms are likely to result in increased bronchorrhea and progressive dyspnea [10]. Large vapor exposure can rapidly produce severe symptoms including seizures, intense bronchorrhea, and apnea leading to death [10]. Severe toxicity from any vapor exposure may occur within minutes of exposure, especially in the case of the nerve agents [10].

Minimal dermal exposures to liquid OPCs may cause only diaphoresis or muscle fasciculations at the site of contact [30]. Minimal and moderate dermal exposures to the nerve agents may cause delayed onset of symptoms (up to 18 hours) due to delayed absorption [30]. Larger dermal exposures can produce systemic symptoms within minutes [30].

Although mydriasis can be seen as a result of nicotinic stimulation, miosis typically predominates in both OPP and nerve agent exposures [2,29]. Miosis was the most common sign among both the primarily exposed patients in Tokyo (99% of patients), in Matsumoto (56%), and secondarily exposed hospital workers [4,9,17,33]. Pupils may be fixed with pupillary reflexes remaining undetectable for days and not returning to normal for weeks [18].

Respiratory system dysfunction is the primary cause of death from both OPPs and nerve agents [15,31,34,35]. Intense bronchorrhea and bronchoconstriction can lead to ventilatory difficulty, refractory hypoxia, and mucus airway obstruction. Nicotinic receptor overstimulation can lead to respiratory muscle fatigue and paralysis. Respiratory failure may occur due to central apnea even before respiratory muscle paralysis (nicotinic) or bronchorrhea (muscarinic) in severe poisoning [31,34]. In the 1995 Tokyo attack, two patients with respiratory arrests and seizures were fully conscious after resuscitation, but unable to breathe on their own [5].

The cardiovascular effects from OPCs are not as predictable as the effects seen in other organ systems. Bradycardia is seen in animals exposed to nerve agents and clinically in humans after severe OPP poisonings [29,36,37], although tachycardia and normal heart rates may also occur [4,5,9,16,38]. Although both hyper- or hypotension can be seen after poisoning, it is interesting to note that the patients from the recent Tokyo attacks had neither [5,9,30,38]. Prolongation of cardiac depolarization and repolarization may occur and may be measured on electrocardiogram as increased length of the measured PR and QT intervals, respectively, when compared to normal values [32,39,40]. Cardiac ischemia may occur as evidenced on electrocardiogram by ST segment changes [32,39]. Dysrhythmias such as ventricular tachycardia and torsades de pointes have also been seen in patients exposed to OPCs [32,39,40].

Signs and symptoms within the gastrointestinal and genitourinary tract range from urinary frequency and loose stools to frank incontinence and copious diarrhea. Nausea and vomiting were common findings in the Tokyo patients [9].

Marked fatigueability is common, and seen early in mild to moderate poisoning [16,41]. Fasciculations and excessive twitching followed by fatigue and flaccid paralysis are seen as the individual muscle fibers, followed by groups of fibers, are overstimulated [10,30].

Giddiness, anxiety, excessive dreaming, forgetfulness, and emotional liability are described with mild to moderate exposure to OPCs [10,15,16]. More significant exposure can result in tremor, paresthesias, seizures, decreased level of consciousness, and headaches [15,16,29,38]. Significant exposure can cause loss of consciousness and centrally mediated apnea [31,34]. Although seizures are reported with significant OPC exposures, electroencephalogram (EEG) abnormalities can be seen without frank seizure activity in the days after even mild intoxications with nerve agents [9,16,38].

Differential diagnosis

The recent sarin experience in Japan demonstrated that patient presentations may not be self-evident, and forensic investigations yielding the correct identity of an agent may be delayed for hours if not days [4,41]. Toxicity from OPCs may be clinically indistinguishable from one another or from exposure to similar compounds, such as carbamate pesticides. Initial treatment, however, is similar, making immediate differentiation less important than recognition of the toxidrome. Cholinomimetic substances such as muscarine containing plants (eg, the jack-o-lantern plant) or the *Inocybe* or *Clitocybe* mushrooms can mimic a muscarinic, cholinergic crisis induced by OPCs [2]. Nicotine containing substances like cigarettes or the *Nicotiana* plant can present with nicotininc overstimulation signs and symptoms.

Chlorine, ammonia, phosgene, or riot control agents may produce dyspnea, lacrimation, and rhinorrhea, but would not be expected to cause the gastrointestinal and urinary symptoms characteristic of cholinergic excess nor the weakness characteristic of nicotinic overstimulation [42]. The erythema and blistering characteristic of vesicant exposure would not be seen with OPCs, although both could cause respiratory and ocular irritation [14,42]. Hydrogen sulfide and cyanide can produce large numbers of seriously ill victims, but the typical cholinergic effects would be absent [42].

Estimate of number of critical care patients

The number of critically ill patients resulting from an OPC attack would greatly depend on factors such as route of dissemination, amount, concentration, location, and route of exposure. St. Luke's Hospital in Tokyo received 640 patients the day of the 1995 sarin attack, many of whom bypassed closer hospitals [42,43]. A single hospital was overwhelmed with patients due to an overall lack of coordination between ambulances and patients bypassing emergency medical services [43]. Only 107 out of the 640 who presented were admitted to the hospital. Five of those were considered critically ill upon presentation; one died in the emergency department and the other four were admitted to the intensive care unit (ICU) [9]. This experience demonstrates that there is little control over when and how patients will present. The Tokyo experience should reemphasize that, just as the emergency department became overwhelmed, the ICU could also, depending on the specific characteristics of a terrorist attack. Therefore, the importance of pre-event planning for surge capability cannot be emphasized enough.

Decontamination

Decontamination is vital to minimize ongoing exposure to victims and to prevent secondary contamination to rescue and medical personnel. Decontamination should be performed outside of the emergency department by trained and properly equipped personnel wearing appropriate personal protective equipment before patient entry into the hospital. Secondary exposure to non- or incompletely decontaminated patients may result in toxicity and health care worker illness and incapacitation [17,44]. Extent and type of decontamination (wet versus dry) will depend on the individual agent and physical/chemical properties. After proper decontamination, universal precautions should always be followed.

In general, decontamination after isolated vapor exposure to very volatile compounds such as sarin should consist of removal of all clothing and jewelry. Failure to remove clothing can result in release of pockets of trapped vapor when patients are undressed in a clinical setting. Physicians at one Japanese hospital became symptomatic during the treatment of sarin poisoned patients from the 1995 Tokyo attack, and several required antidotal therapy [17]. The ventilation of the resuscitation bay, the sealing of patient belongings in vinyl bags, and removal to outside the emergency room halted symptom progression, and no new illness occurred [17]. Additional decontamination methods such as the use of soap and water can be used, but is probably not necessary in these situations. However, if a chemical is placed in a solvent or liquid and then sprayed on victims directly, significant amounts of chemical may remain on the skin. Decontamination with soap and water would therefore be advisable [21].

Decontamination after exposure to liquids or a visible agent should consist of removal of patient clothing and irrigation with copious amounts of water and gentle skin blotting. Scrubbing should be avoided, as this can cause small breaks in the skin and encourage absorption. The addition of a soap solution may enhance decontamination, although copious water alone can be used [21]. Ocular contamination should include copious irrigation with water or saline.

Isolation is only necessary if a patient has not been adequately decontaminated, and only until decontamination, as needed, occurs. If an area of contamination is detected, that is, an exposed patient is sent to the ICU with their original clothing still on, decontamination should occur as rapidly as possible by personnel in appropriate personal protective equipment and at a site remote from other patients to prevent secondary contamination.

Diagnostic studies

The ideal laboratory study for quantification of OPC poisoning would be measurement of active AChE at the neuronal synapse and comparison to a known baseline. As this is not practically possible, surrogate markers including plasma cholinesterase (plasma ChE), erythrocyte cholinesterase (RBC ChE), and population-based reference ranges can be used. Neither alternative marker behaves identically to nervous system AchE; therefore, certain limitations, which impact interpretation, exist.

Plasma ChE is produced by the liver, and activity can be affected by multiple other factors such as pregnancy, medications, infections, and underlying medical illnesses, and even varies in the same person up to 50% when measured over time [15,34,45]. Plasma ChE activity values rapidly fall after exposure to OPCs and, in the case of nerve agent exposure, can rebound to near normal rapidly at times before the patient's symptoms returns to baseline [5,16]. RBC ChE activity is more closely correlated to nervous system AChE than plasma ChE [2,29]. As such, it serves as a more accurate marker of nervous system AChE activity. It, too, would be expected to decline within minutes to hours of OPC exposure depending on the route and dose [16,29]. RBC ChE relies upon erythrocyte turnover to restore normal values at a rate of approximately 1% of baseline per day [16,29,35]. This is considerably slower than nervous system AChE regeneration rates. Therefore, nervous system AChE activity recovery and resolution of cholinergic symptoms may precede "normalization" of EC activity [2,16,29]. Victims of the Tokyo and Matsumoto sarin experiences had initially low PC activity that returned to "normal" within days; however, RBC ChE activity took months to normalize [9,38]. RBC and plasma ChE also have a wide "normal" value range. Patients may have a significant exposure to an AChE inhibitor with a significant drop in cholinesterase activity values, but not fall below the "normal" range [9,35,46]. Furthermore, individual OPCs may affect plasma ChE and RBC ChE differently [15,47].

Severity of illness generally correlates experimentally and clinically with the degree of cholinesterase level decline [16,29,35]. This is not, however, an absolute rule, as some Tokyo patients had equivalently low cholinesterase levels with different degrees of clinical illness [9]. Ocular and dermal exposures that lead to only local effects can produce a significant decrease in cholinesterase levels [14,18]. Other reported abnormal laboratory studies include decreased levels of triglycerides, potassium, chloride, and increased levels of serum creatine kinase, leukocytes, and urine ketones and albumin [9,15,38].

A patient presenting with a cholinergic toxidrome and low levels of cholinesterase activity is usually enough to confirm diagnosis. If further, specific testing is needed to identify the actual etiologic agent, the assistance of specialized research or government labs may be needed. However, results are not likely to be available in a timely fashion to assist clinical management [4]. Nerve agents can be definitively detected and identified for confirmation and public health purposes by sending 25 mL of urine to the regional public health laboratory as described at on the Centers for Disease Control and Prevention Web site [48,49]. Local and state law enforcement, public health, and federal government representatives should be contacted if assistance with definitive testing is required.

Antidote

The overarching goals of antidotal therapy in treating AChE inhibitor poisonings are to control bronchorrhea with antimuscarinic agents, provide oxime therapy before aging occurs (for OPCs), and prevent or terminate seizure activity. Atropine, pralidoxime, and diazepam are the preferred treatments to achieve these goals in the United States. These three agents are also given as autoinjector kits to military personnel for field treatment after nerve agent exposure. The MARK I kit is comprised of atropine (2 mg) and pralidoxime (600 mg) with diazepam dosed as a separate autoinjector [10].

Atropine acts as a competitive antagonist at muscarinic cholinergic receptors in the central and peripheral nervous system. Atropine administration can effectively reverse the muscarinic symptoms of ACh overstimulation seen with AChE inhibitor poisoning in a dose-dependent manner [50]. Atropine has no effect on nicotinic sites and, therefore, exerts no effect on nicotinic symptoms such as muscle weakness, paralysis, fasciculations, or tremor. Atropine may, however, have a role in terminating seizure activity, although it is unclear if it can act to prevent seizures [51–53]. The initial adult dose is 2 mg (0.05 mg/kg in children) intravenously (IV) or intramuscularly (IM) unless the patient is severely poisoned with nerve agents, in which case some authors recommend a larger, up to 6 mg, initial dose in adults [2,21]. Control of bronchorrhea is the endpoint of atropine therapy. Atropine should be redosed at 2- to 5-minute increments until secretions have diminished, airway pressure has decreased, and ventilation is adequate [2,21]. Poisoning resulting from ingestion of OPPs may require hundreds of milligrams of atropine and a continuous infusion to gain control of bronchorrhea [2]. However, in severe military grade nerve agent poisoning, the total dose required over the first several hours may be less than 20 mg [21]. Repeat doses or continuous intravenous infusions may be needed for relapsing symptoms [2,5,29].

Mydriasis and tachycardia should not be used as endpoints to therapy. If ocular absorption of a nerve agent has occurred, miosis may not respond to systemic atropine therapy and can falsely imply continued systemic poisoning long after life-threatening signs of cholinergic excess have resolved [5]. Mydriasis can be treated with a topical long-acting antimuscarinic ophthalmic agent. Tachycardia can occur through either nicotinic stimulation or as a result of distress, fear, or hypoxia. Tachycardia in the setting of continued muscarinic excess (eg, copious respiratory secretions, bronchoconstriction, incontinence) should not be considered a contraindication to atropine use [54].

Multiple casualties resulting from a terrorist attack with an OPC may rapidly deplete in-date, premixed atropine stores. Numerous studies have shown the feasibility, stability, and cost effectiveness of rapid reconstitution of atropine from powder during a mass casualty incident [55–57]. Atropine solutions well past their expiration date still contain significant quantities of atropine [58]. Diphenhydramine, as a second line agent, may be of some benefit because it crosses the blood–brain barrier [34]. Glycopyrrolate, ipratropium, and other antimuscarinics that do not cross the blood–brain barrier would not be expected to ameliorate the central effects of OPC poisoning, and should not be used as mono-therapy, although certain circumstances may benefit from their use as adjuncts to atropine therapy [2,34]. Glycopyrrolate may be effective in treating isolated peripheral muscarinic signs, particularly in patients who develop excessive central antimuscarinic syndromes from atropine therapy [2]. Nebulized ipratropium may help treat pulmonary muscarinic symptoms when used in conjunction with systemic atropine therapy [2].

The oxime compounds are AChE reactivators that act by breaking the bond between AChE and the nerve agent, thus freeing AChE to degrade ACh. This is only possible before the aging process is complete. The action of oximes occurs most markedly at nicotinic sites (neuromuscular junction) and acts in synergy with atropine [2,20].

Pralidoxime, the oxime approved for use in the United States, is a quaternary nitrogen compound. As such, it has limited ability to cross the blood–brain barrier, although there are human case reports that suggest some CNS penetration [20,29,59].

The optimal dosing regimen of pralidoxime for OPC poisoning is unknown. The generally recommended initial dose is 1 to 2 g for adults (25–50 mg/kg in children) given IV over 15 to 30 minutes [60–64]. The half-life of pralidoxime is less than 80 minutes when administered either IV or IM, making it theoretically difficult to maintain adequate blood levels without either frequent redosing or continuous infusions [62,63,65]. It is unclear as to whether repeat bolus dosing or a continuous infusion is the optimal pralidoxime dosing regimen for nerve agent exposures. However, logic and clinical evidence suggests a continuous infusion would be more effective due to the avoidance of normal concentration peaks and troughs encountered with repeat bolus dosing [62,63]. Data suggests that a minimum level of 4 μg/mL is needed to antagonize nicotinic symptoms, although even higher serum concentrations may be needed [66–68]. Most authors recommend an intravenous infusion in adults that can be titrated to effect at 200 to 500 mg/h (5–20 mg/kg/h in children) [60–63]. If a drip is not started, repeat dosing should be considered every 3 to 8 hours for signs of poisoning [5,69]. Rapid bolus dosing or infusions at greater than 200 mg/min should be avoided, as these can produce significant symptoms including cardiac or respiratory arrest [20,21,60,61]. Pralidoxime may require dosing adjustment in renally impaired patients [70]. Other oxime compounds such as obidoxime and HI-6 exist, and have agent-dependent affinities [71].

Benzodiazepines, such as diazepam, should be used for control of seizures. In the hospital setting, diazepam is recommended in initial doses of 5 to 10 mg IV for seizure control [10,21]. Although atropine may have some role in the treatment of OPC-induced seizures, diazepam or another benzodiazepine should be used as a first-line agent to terminate seizure activity and preserve neurological function [52,53]. Diazepam may exacerbate OPC-induced respiratory depression; therefore, a patient's airway and mental status should be monitored carefully during therapy [21]. Animal studies suggest that diazepam, in conjunction with OPC antidotal therapy, can actually inhibit organophosphate-induced central respiratory depression, prevent neuropathic damage, and improve outcome [72,73]. Antiepileptic agents such as fosphenytoin have no role in terminating nerve agent-induced seizures [74].

Pyridostigmine is a reversible carbamate-type AChE inhibitor. Its use as a pretreatment agent for partial protection against possible future OPC poisoning in conjunction with traditional therapy has been suggested. The theoretical reasoning behind this therapy is that some AChE (minimal) would be inhibited by pyridostigmine before OPC exposure. Because pyridostigmine reversibly binds to AChE, if a real OPC exposure occurred, pyridostigmine bound AChE would be unavailable for binding. After the acute event, the pyridostigmine–AChE complexes will disassociate, because aging does not occur with carbamates. This will leave a portion of the patient's overall AChE activity intact. The true battlefield efficacy of this idea has yet to be definitively determined. There is no indication for pyridostigmine treatment of patients who have already been exposed and therapy for victims who have been pretreated with pyridostigmine does not differ.

Supportive care

As respiratory failure is usually the cause of death in OPC poisoning, aggressive ventilatory support including endotracheal intubation should be considered early. If rapid sequence intubation is performed, succinylcholine, although not absolutely contraindicated, should be avoided if possible. Succinylcholine is metabolized by plasma ChE, and OPC-induced inhibition can lead to prolonged neuromuscular blockade [75,76]. Intubations may be complicated by excessive secretions, so the operator is advised to prepare for aggressive suctioning and for the possibility of an emergency surgical airway. Maintenance of adequate ventilation may be complicated by mucus plugging and bronchoconstriction; therefore, continued suctioning, along with antidotal therapy, should be performed to minimize airway obstruction.

General supportive care also includes cardiac and neurologic monitoring as well as maintenance and monitoring of fluid status. Crystalloid fluid resuscitation may be needed, as excessive secretions can cause volume depletion. Continuous cardiac monitoring should be performed with regular assessment of PR and QT intervals by electrocardiogram. Continuous, or at least frequent, EEG monitoring may be beneficial to detect epileptiform activity in a chemically paralyzed patient. Seizures should be treated aggressively with drug-induced anticonvulsant medications like the benzodiazepine and barbiturate class of medications.

Appropriate radiologic studies should be performed promptly to diagnose treatable conditions (eg, subdural, epidural) or assist in determining prognosis (eg, evidence of severe hypoxic injury) as needed. Prolonged need for ventilatory support may be required with significant OPP exposures, but lack of significant improvement with antidote therapy should prompt the clinician to look for underlying traumatic or hypoxic injury from either prolonged periods of hypoventilation, seizure activity or head trauma.

Clinical course and prognostic factors

Symptom onset is likely to begin within minutes after a nerve agent exposure through any route including dermal contact if the exposure is large enough [10,77,78]. Exposure to nerve agent vapors are very likely to cause symptoms within minutes [10]. Certain highly lipid soluble OPCs such as fenthion and chlorfenthion may delay symptom onset to more than 12 hours after contact. Ingestion of most OPCs and nerve agents are likely to cause rapid onset of symptoms, although VX consumption may delay symptom onset by several hours [10,47].

The duration of OPC toxicity is dependent on the type of agent, lipid solubility, route of exposure, and dose. The Japanese experience with the diluted, poorly disseminated sarin subway incident found that even critically ill patients were able to be weaned off the ventilator within 1 to 2 days and discharged from the hospital within a week with the exception of a single patient, who also suffered severe hypoxemic brain damage [9]. However, the circumstances of this situation and small numbers of critically ill patients severely limit large-scale extrapolation of findings. Very lipophillic pesticides such as dichlofenthion may cause persistent cholinergic effects for several days [79].

Intermediate syndrome, a poorly understood phenomenon, may occur in some OPP poisoned patients, but has not been documented after nerve agent exposures [80,81]. It usually occurs between 24 and 96 hours after initial clinical improvement, which may include return of consciousness and extubation. Affected patients can develop neck, trunk, and proximal extremity muscle weakness to the point of paralysis [80,81]. These patients can also develop decreased levels of consciousness, decreased reflexes, and require reintubation with days to weeks of ventilatory support [80,81]. Supportive care, reinstitution of pralidoxime therapy, and atropine, if needed to control muscarinic toxicity, is indicated [2,80,81].

Certain effects may persist after recovery from acute OPC toxicity. Miosis may persist for weeks after OPC poisoning [18]. Minimal EEG and electrocardiogram changes were present in after a year in more than half of a group of severely sarin-exposed patients from Matsumoto, Japan [82]. Peripheral neuropathies are reported after severe OPP poisoning [7,83]. The etiology is thought to be inhibition of an enzyme in neuronal tissue known as neuropathy target esterase, which leads to an axonopathy [84,85]. There have been some reports of neuropathy in patients after the sarin exposures in Japan, although the etiology and the extent is not clear [38,86]. Increased rates of sister chromatid changes suggest there may be genotoxic effects from nerve agent exposure, although resultant carcinogenic effects are unknown [87].

Prognosis

Prolonged periods of hypoxia and seizures are the most influential factors on a patient's prognosis after an OPC exposure [9,53]. Once aging occurs, bound enzyme is functionally inactive and the patient must synthesize new AChE. Available evidence supports that in nerve agent toxicity, most patients respond well to antidote therapy if administered rapidly enough, in conjunction with basic supportive care, and have relatively brief requirements for intensive care support. OPC exposures can require considerably longer hospital stays, during which typical ICU complications such as infections can impact a patient's prognosis.

Summary

Nerve agents and OPP exposures must be recognized early and treated aggressively. Early airway and ventilatory support should occur in conjunction with antidotal therapy. Atropine should be titrated to control bronchorrhea. Initial pralidoxime therapy should be given as soon as possible in suspected OPC poisoning and ideally before aging occurs. Successful therapy for OPC poisoning may include repeat dosing of pralidoxime or a continuous infusion, depending on the situation. Diazepam should be given to control seizures that may occur in severe poisoning. Late complications depend on the type of OPC involved, and can include intermediate syndrome and peripheral neuropathy.

References

[1] Organisation for the Prohibition of Chemical Weapons. The chemical weapons ban: facts and figures. Available at www.opcw.org/factsandfigures/html/ff_print.html. Last accessed March 26, 2005.
[2] Clark RF. Insecticides: organic phosphorus compounds and carbamates. In: Goldfrank LR, Flomenbaum NE, Lewin NA, Howland MA, Hoffman RS, Nelson LS, editors. Goldfrank's toxicologic emergencies. 7th edition. New York: McGraw-Hill; 2002. p. 1346–60.
[3] Smart JK. History of chemical and biological warfare: an American perspective. In: Sidell FR, Takafuji ET, Franz DR, editors. Medical aspects of chemical and biological warfare (Textbook of military medicine, part I: warfare weaponry, and the casualty). Washington (DC): Office of the Surgeon General; 1997. p. 9–86.
[4] Okudera H. Clinical feature on nerve gas terrorism in Matsumoto. J Clin Neurosci 2002;9(1): 17–21.
[5] Ohbu S, Yamashina A, Takasu N, et al. Sarin poisoning on Tokyo subway. South Med J 1997; 90(6):587–93.
[6] De Letter EA, Cordonnier JACM, Piette MHA. An unusual case of homicide by use of repeated administration of organophosphate insecticides. J Clin Forensic Med 2002;9:15–21.

[7] Moretto A, Lotti M. Poisoning by organophosphorous insecticides and sensory neuropathy. J Neurol Neurosurg Psychiatry 1998;64:463–8.

[8] Wu ML, Deng JF, Tsai WJ, et al. Food poisoning due to methamidophos-contaminated vegetables. J Toxicol Clin Toxicol 2001;34(4):333–6.

[9] Okumura T, Takasu N, Ishimatsu S, et al. Report on 640 victims of the Tokyo subway sarin attack. Ann Emerg Med 1996;28(2):129–35.

[10] Sidell FR. Nerve agents. In: Sidell FR, Takafuji ET, Franz DR, editors. Medical aspects of chemical and biological warfare (Textbook of military medicine, part I: warfare weaponry, and the casualty). Washington (DC): Office of the Surgeon General; 1997. p. 129–79.

[11] Greenaway C, Orr P. A foodborne outbreak causing a cholinergic syndrome. J Emerg Med 1996; 14(3):339–44.

[12] CDC. Recognition of illness associated with exposure to chemical agents – United States, 2003. MMWR Morb Mortal Wkly Rep 2003;52(39):938–40.

[13] EXTOXNET. Pesticide information profiles. Available at http://etoxnet.orst.edu/pips/ghindex. html. Last accessed March 26, 2005.

[14] Craig FN, Cummings EG, Sim VM. Environmental temperature and the percutaneous absorption of a cholinesterase inhibitor, VX. J Invest Dermatol 1977;68:357–61.

[15] Gallo MA, Lawryk NJ. Organic phosphorus pesticides. In: Hayes WJ, Laws ER, editors. Classes of pesticides, volume 2 (Handbook of pesticide toxicology). New York: Academic Press, Inc.; 1991. p. 917–1123.

[16] Grob D, Harvey JC. Effects in man of the anticholinesterase compound sarin (isopropyl methyl phosphonofluridate). J Clin Invest 1958;37(3):350–68.

[17] Nozaki H, Hori S, Shinozawa Y, et al. Secondary exposure of medical staff to sarin vapor in the emergency room. Intensive Care Med 1995;21:1032–5.

[18] Rengstorff RH. Accidental exposure to sarin: vision effects. Arch Toxiol 1985;56:201–3.

[19] Hoffman BB, Taylor P. Neurotransmission: the autonomic and somatic motor nervous system. In: Hardman JG, Limbird LE, Gilman AG, editors. Goodman & Gilman's the pharmacological basis of therapeutics. 10th edition. New York: McGraw Hill; 2001. p. 115–54.

[20] Taylor P. Anticholinesterase agents. In: Hardman JG, Limbird LE, Gilman AG, editors. Goodman & Gilman's the pharmacological basis of therapeutics. 10th edition. New York: McGraw Hill; 2001. p. 175–92.

[21] Sidell FR, Borak J. Chemical warfare agents: II. Nerve agents. Ann Emerg Med 1991;21(7): 865–71.

[22] Mason HJ, Waine E, Stevenson A, et al. Aging and spontaneous reactivation of human plasma cholinesterase activity after inhibition by organophosphorus pesticides. Hum Exp Toxicol 1993; 12(6):497–503.

[23] Masson P, Goasdoue JL. Evidence that the conformational stability of "aged" organophosphate-inhibited cholinesterase is altered. Biochem Biophys Acta 1986;869(3):304–13.

[24] Rotenberg M, Shefi M, Dany S, et al. Differentiation between organophosphate and carbamate poisoning. Clin Chim Acta 1995;234(1–2):11–21.

[25] Gant DB, Eldefrawi ME, Eldefrawi AT. Action of organophosphates on $GABA_A$ receptor and voltage dependent chloride channels. Fundam Appl Toxicol 1987;9:698–704.

[26] Liu DD, Watanabe HK, Ho IK, et al. Acute effects of soman, sarin, and tabun on cyclic nucleotide metabolism in rat striatum. J Toxicol Environ Health 1986;19(1):23–32.

[27] Tang HW, Cassel G. Effect of soman on N-methyl-D-aspartate-stimulated [^{3}H]norepinephrine release from rat cortical slices. Toxicol Lett 1998;99(3):169–73.

[28] Silveira CL, Eldefrawi AT, Elderfrawi ME. Putative M2 muscarinic receptors of rat heart have high affinity for organophosphorous anticholinesterases. Toxicol Appl Pharmacol 1990; 103:474–81.

[29] Namba T, Nolte CT, Jackrel J, et al. Poisoning due to organophosphate insecticides. Am J Med 1971;50:475–92.

[30] Sidell FR. Clinical considerations in nerve agents intoxication. In: Somani SM, editor. Chemical warfare agents. New York: Academic Press Inc.; 1992. p. 156–94.

[31] Rickett DL, Glenn JF, Beers ET. Central respiratory effects versus neuromuscular actions of nerve agents. Neurotoxicology 1986;7(1):225–36.

[32] Saadeh AM, Farasakh NA, Al-Ali MK. Cardiac manifestations of acute carbamate and organophosphate poisoning. Heart 1997;77:461–4.

[33] Okudera H, Morita H, Iwashita T, et al. Unexpected nerve gas exposure in the city of Matsumoto: report of rescue activity in the first sarin gas terrorism. Am J Emerg Med 1997; 15(5):527–8.

[34] Bird SB, Gaspari RJ, Dickson EW. Early death due to severe organophosphate poisoning is a centrally mediated process. Acad Emerg Med 2003;10(4):295–8.

[35] Slapper D. Toxicity, organophosphate and carbamate. Available at www.emedicine.com/emerg/topic246.htm. Last accessed on March 29, 2005.

[36] Chang FCT, Gouty SC, Eder LC, et al. Cardiorespiratory effects of O-Isobutyl S-[2-(diethylamino)-ethyl] methylphosphonothioate—a structural isomer of VX. J Appl Toxicol 1998;18:337–47.

[37] Lifshitz M, Shahak E, Sofer S. Carbamate and organophosphate poisoning in young children. Pediatr Emerg Care 1999;15(2):102–3.

[38] Morita H, Yanagisawa N, Nakajima T, et al. Sarin poisoning in Matsumoto, Japan. Lancet 1995;346:290–3.

[39] Karki P, Ansari JA, Koirala BS. Cardiac and electrocardiographical manifestations of acute organophosphate poisoning. Singapore Med J 2004;45(8):385–9.

[40] Ludomirsky A, Klein HO, Sarelli P, et al. Q-T prolongation and polymorphous ("Torsade de Pointes") ventricular arrhythmias associated with organophosphorus insecticide poisoning. Am J Cardiol 1982;49:1654–8.

[41] Okumura T, Suzuki K, Fukuda A, et al. The Tokyo subway sarin attack: disaster management, part 2: hospital response. Acad Emerg Med 1998;5(6):618–24.

[42] CDC. Case definitions for chemical poisoning. MMWR Recomm Rep 2005;54(RR-1):1–24.

[43] Okumura T, Suzuki K, Fukuda A, et al. The Tokyo subway sarin attack: disaster management, part 1: community emergency response. Acad Emerg Med 1998;5(6):613–7.

[44] CDC. Nosocomial poisoning associated with emergency department treatment of organophosphate toxicity—Georgia 2000. MMWR Morb Mortal Wkly Rep 2001;49(51):1156–8.

[45] Sidell FR, Kaminskis A. Temporal intrapersonal physiological variability of cholinesterase activity in human plasma and erythrocytes. Clin Chem 1975;21(13):1961–3.

[46] Coye MJ, Barnett PG, Midtling JE, et al. Clinical confirmation of organophosphate poisoning by serial cholinesterase analyses. Arch Intern Med 1987;147:438–42.

[47] Sidell FR, Groff WA. The reactivatability of cholinesterase inhibited by VX and sarin in man. Toxicol Appl Pharm 1974;27:241–52.

[48] CDC. Shipping instructions for specimens collected from people potentially exposed to chemical terrorism agents. Available at http://www.bt.cdc.gov/labissues/pdf/shipping-samples.pdf. Last accessed May 4, 2005.

[49] CDC. Chemical terrorism event specimen collection. Available at http://www.bt.cdc.gov/labissues/pdf/chemspecimencollection.pdf. Last accessed May 4, 2005.

[50] Brown JH, Taylor P. Muscarinic receptor agonists and antagonists. In: Hardman JG, Limbird LE, Gilman AG, editors. Goodman & Gilman's the pharmacological basis of therapeutics. 10th edition. New York: McGraw Hill; 2001. p. 155–74.

[51] McDonough JH, Zoeffel LD, McMonagle J, et al. Anticonvulsant treatment of nerve agent seizures: anticholinergics versus diazepam in soman-intoxicated guinea pigs. Epilepsy Res 2000; 38:1–14.

[52] Shih TM, McDonough JH. Organophosphorus nerve agents-induced seizures and efficacy of atropine sulfate as anticonvulsant treatment. Pharmacol Biochem Behav 1999;64(1):147–53.

[53] Shih TM, Duniho SM, McDonough JH. Control of nerve agent-induced seizures is critical for neuroprotection and survival. Toxicol Appl Pharm 2003;188:69–80.

[54] Dunn MA, Sidell FR. Progress in medical defense against nerve agents. JAMA 1989;262(5): 649–52.

[55] Dix J, Weber RJ, Frye RE, et al. Stability of atropine sulfate prepared for mass chemical terrorism. J Toxicol Clin Toxicol 2003;41(6):771–5.

[56] Geller RJ, Lopez GP, Cutler S, et al. Atropine availability as an antidote for nerve agent casualties: validated rapid reformulation of high-concentration atropine from bulk powder. Ann Emerg Med 2003;41(4):453–6.

[57] Kosak RJ, Deigel S, Kuzma J. Rapid atropine synthesis for the treatment of massive nerve agent exposure. Ann Emerg Med 2003;41(5):685–8.

[58] Schier JG, Ravikumar PR, Nelson LS, et al. Preparing for chemical terrorism: stability of injectable atropine sulfate. Acad Emerg Med 2004;11(4):329–34.

[59] Lotti M, Becker C. Treatment of acute organophosphate-poisoning: evidence of a direct effect on central nervous systems by 2-PAM (Pyridine-2-aldoxime methyl chloride). J Toxicol Clin Toxicol 1982;19:121–7.

[60] Geller RJ. Pralidoxime (2-PAM) and other oximes. In: Olson KR, Anderson IB, Benowitz NL, Blanc PD, Clark RF, Kearney TE, et al, editors. Poisoning & drug overdose. 4th edition. New York: McGraw Hill; 2004. p. 492–4.

[61] Howland MA. Antidotes in depth: pralidoxime. In: Goldfrank LR, Flomenbaum NE, Lewin NA, Howland MA, Hoffman RS, Nelson LS, editors. Goldfrank's toxicologic emergencies. 7th ed. New York: McGraw-Hill; 2002. p. 1361–5.

[62] Medicus JJ, Stork CM, Howland MA, et al. Pharmacokinetics following a loading plus a continuous infusion of pralidoxime compared with the traditional short infusion regimen in human volunteers. J Toxicol Clin Toxicol 1996;34(3):289–95.

[63] Schexnayder S, James LP, Kearns GL, et al. The pharmacokinetics of continuous infusion pralidoxime in children with organophosphate poisoning. J Toxicol Clin Toxicol 1998;36(6): 549–55.

[64] Singh S, Chaudhry D, Behera D, et al. Aggressive atropinization and continuous pralidoxime (2-PAM) infusion in patients with severe organophosphate poisoning: experience of a northwest Indian hospital. Hum Exp Toxicol 2001;20:15–8.

[65] Sidell FR, Groff WA. Intramuscular and intravenous administration of small doses of –Pyridium aldoxime methochloride to man. J Pharm Sci 1971;60(8):1224–8.

[66] Sundwall A. Minimal concentration of N-Methlpyriinium-2-Aldoxime methane sulphonate (P2S) which reverse neuromuscular block. Biochem Pharmacol 1961;8:413–7.

[67] Thompson DF, Thompson GD, Greenwood RB, et al. Therapeutic dosing of pralidoxime chloride. Drug Intell Clin Pharm 1987;21:590–3.

[68] Worek F, Backer M, Thiermann H, et al. Reappraisal of indications and limitations of oxime therapy in organophosphate poisoning. Hum Exp Toxicol 1997;16:466–72.

[69] Tush GM, Anstead MI. Pralidoxime continuous infusion in the treatment of organophosphate poisoning. Ann Pharm 1997;31:441–4.

[70] Holstedge CP, Kirk M, Sidell FR. Chemical warfare: nerve agent poisoning. Crit Care Clin 1997;13(4):923–42.

[71] Worek F, Widmann R, Knopff O, et al. Reactivating potency of obidoxime, pralidoxime, HI 6, HLö 7 in human erythrocyte acetylcholinesterase inhibited by highly toxic organophosphorus compounds. Arch Toxicol 1998;72:237–43.

[72] Dickson EW, Bird SB, Gaspari RJ, et al. Diazepam inhibits organophosphate-induced central respiratory depression. Acad Emerg Med 2003;10(12):1303–6.

[73] Tuovinen K. Organophosphate-induced convulsions and prevention of neuropathological damages. Toxicology 2004;196:31–9.

[74] McDonough JH, Benjamin A, McMonagle JD, et al. Effects of fosphenytoin on nerve agent-induced status epilepticus. Drug Chem Toxicol 2004;27(1):27–39.

[75] Seldon BS, Curry SC. Prolonged succinylcholine-induced paralysis in organophosphate insecticide poisoning. Ann Emerg Med 1987;16:215–7.

[76] Sener EB, Ustun E, Kocamanoglu S, et al. Prolonged apnea following succinylcholine administration in undiagnosed acute organophosphate poisoning. Acta Anaesthesiol Scand 2002;46: 1046–8.

[77] Halle A, Sloas DD. Percutaneous organophosphate poisoning. South Med J 1987;80(9): 1179–81.

[78] Lokan R, James R. Rapid death by mevinphos poisoning while under observation. Forensic Sci Int 1983;22(2–3):179–82.

[79] Davies JE, Barquet A, Freed VH, et al. Human pesticide poisonings by a fat-soluble organo-phosphate insecticide. Arch Environ Health 1975;30(12):608–13.

[80] Senanayake N, Karalliedde L. Neurotoxic effects of organophosphorus insecticides: an inter-mediate syndrome. N Engl J Med 1987;316(13):761–3.

[81] Sudakin DL, Mullins ME, Horowitz BZ, et al. Intermediate syndrome after malathion ingestion despite continuous infusion of pralidoxime. J Toxicol Clin Toxicol 2000;38(1):47–50.

[82] Sekijima Y, Morita H, Yanagisawa N. Follow-up of sarin poisoning in Matsumoto. Ann Intern Med 1997;127(11):1042.

[83] Wolff AD. Ginger jake and the blues: a tragic song of poisoning. Vet Hum Toxicol 1995;37(3): 252–4.

[84] Barrett DS, Dehme FW, Kruckenberg SM. A review of organophosphorus ester induced delayed neurotoxicity. Vet Hum Toxicol 1985;27(1):22–37.

[85] Mutch E, Blain PG, Williams FM. Interindividual variations in enzymes controlling organo-phosphate toxicity in man. Hum Exp Toxicol 1992;11(2):109–16.

[86] Himuro K, Murayama S, Nishiyama K, et al. Distal sensory axonopathy after sarin intoxication. Neurology 1998;51(4):1195–7.

[87] Li Q, Hirata Y, Kawada T, et al. Elevated frequency of sister chromatid exchanges of lym-phocytes in sarin-exposed victims of the Tokyo sarin disaster 3 years after the event. Toxicology 2004;201:209–17.

ELSEVIER
SAUNDERS

CRITICAL
CARE
CLINICS

Crit Care Clin 21 (2005) 691–705

Cyanides

Anthony P. Morocco, MD

*Guam Memorial Hospital, Department of Emergency Medicine, 850 Gov. Carlos Camacho Road,
Oka, Tamuning, Guam 96911*

Perhaps no other poison is so universally recognized as cyanide. Since antiquity, the lethality of cyanide-containing plants has been well known. The Roman Emperor Nero dispatched his enemies with cyanogenic cherry laurel water, and other forms of cyanide have since been used by common murderers and militaries alike [1].

Hydrogen cyanide (HCN) was first isolated in 1782 by Scheele, who later died after being poisoned by the substance. The name cyanide is derived from the colorful Prussian blue from which HCN (also called prussic acid) was first synthesized [2]. Massive quantities of cyanides are produced in industry every year, for use in metal extraction, electroplating, pesticides, metal hardening, photography, printing, dyeing, and many other manufacturing processes. In addition, cyanogenic (cyanide-forming) compounds such as amygdalin are naturally occurring in many *Prunus* species seeds and fruit pits, including bitter almonds, apricots, chokeberries, and apples, and in other common food sources such as lima beans and cassava [3]. Cyanides are also produced during the combustion of many organic compounds [4].

Battlefield use of cyanides was proposed by Napoleon III during the Franco-Prussian war, to improve the lethality of bayonets. The French introduced gaseous HCN to World War I in 1915, and used 4000 tons in battle. However, it was found to be a relatively poor weapon due to its poor persistence in open battlefields and difficulty in delivering large amounts in small artillery shells, and the Germans soon equipped their soldiers with gas masks that filtered the cyanide [5]. French attempts at an improved warfare agent resulted in the introduction of cyanogen chloride in 1916, which had the advantages of lower volatility and the ability to cause additional toxicity (mucous membrane irritation and lung injury)

E-mail address: morocco@pobox.com

at lower concentrations. A related compound, cyanogen bromide, was simultaneously introduced by Austria, but was difficult to use and subsequently abandoned. Germany did not use cyanide during the First World War, but it did infamously use HCN, in the form of the fumigant Zyklon B, to exterminate millions of Jews and other prisoners during the Second World War. Japan may have also used cyanide against the Chinese during this era. Cyanide has since been reportedly used in the 1980s in the Iran–Iraq war, against the Kurds in Halabja, and in the Syrian city of Hama [1].

Numerous well-publicized incidents resulting in deaths, both intentional and unintentional, have occurred due to nonmilitary uses of cyanide. A mixture of toxic gases including methyl isocyanate and cyanides was responsible for up to 5000 deaths and 200,000 injuries in the Bhopal, India, chemical plant disaster [6]. In 1978, a cyanide-laced drink was used in the mass suicide of 913 followers of the Reverend Jim Jones in Jonestown, Guyana. Several well-publicized murder plots have involved cyanide-laced food or commercial products, including the adulteration of acetaminophen capsules that killed seven Chicagoans in 1982 [7]. HCN has also been used in the "gas chamber" for prisoner executions in the United States.

Given its notorious history and notoriety as a poison, it is not surprising that terrorists have identified cyanide as a valuable addition to their arsenals. The 1993 World Trade Center bombers may have attempted to incorporate cyanide into their attack. Although the use of sarin nerve agent in the Tokyo subway in 1995 was well publicized, less well known is that containers of cyanide precursors were discovered in subway bathrooms after the attack. More recently, several potential cyanide attacks appear to have been foiled. In 2002, al-Qaeda affiliated terrorists were arrested in connection with plots to release cyanide gas in the London Underground and to poison the water supply at the US embassy in Rome with cyanide. Also, in 2002, a cyanide cache linked to suspected al-Qaeda operatives was found in Paris. In 2003, the captured arsenal of an American White Supremacist group was found to contain cyanide, and a man was convicted of placing bottles of cyanide in train tunnels in Chicago [7].

Mechanism of toxicity

Cyanide compounds, in gaseous, liquid, or solid states, could be used in a number of potential terrorist attack scenarios. Weaponized cyanide has most commonly been in the form of the volatile liquids HCN and cyanogen chloride. HCN is known by the North Atlantic Treaty Organization (NATO) designation AC, while cyanogen chloride is designated CK. The physical properties of such agents are a critical determinant of their effectiveness in a chemical attack. HCN is water soluble, and has a boiling point of 25.7°C (78.3F). It is highly volatile, lighter than air as a vapor, and smells like bitter almonds. Cyanogen chloride boils at 12.9°C (55.2F) but is less volatile and denser than HCN [1]. Cyanide also exists as a number of inorganic salts, including sodium, potassium, and calcium cyanide. The addition of a mineral acid to a cyanide salt results in the liberation of HCN gas [4].

A terrorist attack could involve HCN or cyanogen chloride in a number of ways. Large quantities of both chemicals are readily available, as they are manufactured and transported for industrial use. The most commonly discussed scenario is the release of HCN in an enclosed and crowded space. An outdoor release would require higher quantities of gas and would be less effective due to the dispersion of the gases. The gas could be released from a storage container or could be generated at the site using precursors such as cyanide salts. Adulteration of food or water supplies with a cyanide salt is another potential terrorist scenario. Given cyanide's notoriety as a poison, any intentional release, even a small-scale event, would undoubtedly create an enormous panic with an impact far beyond the number of direct casualties.

The most likely exposure to cyanide during a terrorist event could be an unintended consequence. Historically, the vast majority of attacks have involved conventional explosives and resulting fires. During combustion, nitrogen and carbon-containing substances generate toxic gases including HCN. The burning of natural substances such as paper, cotton, wool, silk, and synthetic plastics and other polymers can release large quantities of HCN. High-temperature and low-oxygen environments, present in enclosed area fires, enhance the degradation of these materials and increase toxic gas production. For example, polyacrylonitrile, a polymer used in numerous fabrics, upholstery covers, and furniture padding, can produce half its mass as HCN upon thermal decomposition [8]. Several investigations have suggested cyanide as an important contributor to fire-related deaths [9–11].

No matter the mechanism of exposure, HCN and cyanogen chloride are quickly absorbed in the lungs and mucous membranes. Significant dermal absorption can occur after exposure to high concentrations of a powdered cyanide salt or aqueous solutions, particularly if the skin integrity is compromised by trauma or burns [4]. HCN is a weak acid, existing primarily as HCN at physiologic pH. This small, nonionized molecule easily moves across cell membranes. Cyanogen chloride rapidly releases cyanide in the body, thus the agents AC and CK will have identical systemic physiologic effects [12].

Cyanide's mechanism of action as a poison is its inhibition of numerous enzyme systems, including xanthine oxidase, carbonic anhydrase, glutamate decarboxylase, and cytochrome oxidase. Binding to the ferric iron of cytochrome a_3, the last enzyme in the mitochondrial electron transport chain, is considered cyanide's most important effect [4,13]. During normal cell energy production, glucose first undergoes glycolysis in the cytoplasm, producing pyruvate and adenosine triphosphate (ATP; Fig. 1). Pyruvate then enters the mitochondrion, where it is used by the tricarboxylic acid cycle in producing electron donors for the oxidative phosphorylation occurring in the mitochondrial inner membrane. It is this electron transport chain, facilitated by the cytochrome oxidase enzyme system, which consumes oxygen and generates the bulk of cellular ATP. Cyanide poisoning inhibits this enzyme system, shutting down the cell's aerobic pro-

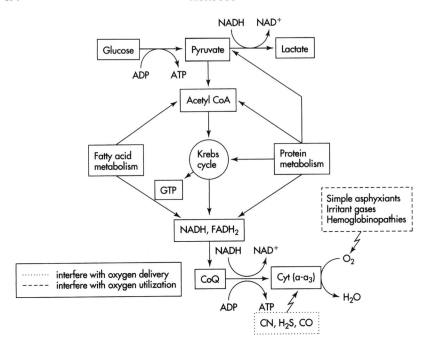

Fig. 1. Mechanism of action of cyanide.

duction of energy. Oxygen consumption is decreased, while glycolysis continues to convert glucose to pyruvate, which is then converted to lactate for relatively inefficient anaerobic ATP production. Systemic acidosis occurs not via lactate production, but through continued hydrogen ion production by cellular use of ATP without the normal balancing hydrogen ion consumption by oxidative phosphorylation [4,14].

The metabolic effects of cyanide poisoning are most pronounced in the brain and cardiovascular system, as any process that impairs oxygen use preferentially affects the most critically ATP-dependent organs first. The development of hypotension and acidosis exacerbates oxygen use and organ dysfunction [4]. The brain and heart are also found to have the highest concentration of cyanide postmortem [4]. Cardiac cytochrome oxidase is particularly sensitive to cyanide [15]. The brain is most affected by cyanide-induced oxidative stress and lipid peroxidation. Cyanide's inhibition of enzymes such as superoxide dismutase, catalase, and glutathione reductase may enhance generation of damaging reactive oxygen species [16].

Cyanide may also cause neurotoxicity through excitatory neurotransmitter effects. Release of glutamate, stimulation of N-methyl-D-aspartate receptors, and enhancement of cytosolic calcium release result in cell death [17]. Dopaminergic neurons of the basal ganglia seem to be most sensitive to this cyanide-induced neurotoxicity [18]. The brain may also be affected by cyanide's inhibition of glutamate decarboxylase, an enzyme responsible for the production of γ-aminobutryic acid (GABA). The loss of GABA's inhibitory effects increases the risk of seizures [19].

Clinical presentation

The clinical presentation of cyanide toxicity varies considerably depending on the cyanide compound, method of exposure, and dose. Signs and symptoms are nonspecific and generally reflect cyanide's central nervous system and cardiovascular effects. Exposures to high doses of HCN or cyanogen chloride gases are rapidly fatal. Estimates of lethal dose vary, but exposures to gaseous HCN at concentrations above 300 parts per million (ppm) will likely result in death within a few minutes, while concentrations of 100 ppm could be fatal after 30 to 60 minutes. Oral doses of 50 mg of HCN or 200 to 300 mg of potassium cyanide are likely to be fatal [4,13]. Upon exposure to high concentrations of HCN gas, patients quickly develop hyperpnea (within 15 seconds) and loss of consciousness (within 30 seconds). Within 3 to 5 minutes apnea occurs, followed by loss of cardiac activity and death 5 to 8 minutes after exposure. Lower concentrations result in a more prolonged course of signs and symptoms. Patients develop dyspnea, headache, weakness, nausea, vomiting, dizziness, flushing, anxiety, and an altered level of consciousness. Central nervous system toxicity may then advance to seizures and coma with diminished pupillary response [1]. Cardiovascular toxicity manifests as early hypertension and tachycardia, followed by progressive bradycardia, atrioventricular block, ventricular arrhythmias, and finally asystole [4].

Exposure to cyanogen chloride differs from HCN in that patients will complain of significant eye and mucous membrane irritation upon exposure. After low-dose exposures, patients present with lacrimation, rhinorrhea, and bronchorrhea. Chest tightness, cough, and shortness of breath can also occur due to lung injury and pulmonary edema [12]. Higher doses cause the same systemic toxicity as HCN exposure. Ingestion of cyanide salts causes an identical clinical picture, but symptoms may be delayed 15 to 30 minutes, while symptoms can occur hours after ingestion of naturally occurring cyanogenic compounds and nitriles that require biotransformation to liberate cyanide. The corrosive nature of alkaline aqueous cyanide solutions and cyanide salts can also cause significant skin burns and gastrointestinal tract injury in addition to the systemic toxicity. After oral ingestion, patients will develop nausea, vomiting, and abdominal pain [4,13].

One potentially important physical finding is the bitter almond odor of HCN as the gas is excreted from the patient's lungs. Unfortunately, only 40% to 60% of the population is capable of detecting this odor, with a wide variation of odor threshold and rapid olfactory fatigue [4,20]. Other findings can include a cherry red color to the skin, as well as similar color appearance of retinal veins and arteries [21]. Impairment of oxygen use may result in bright red venous blood due to an elevated venous oxygen saturation. Patients can instead appear cyanotic due to apnea and shock [4].

A patient with an unknown cyanide exposure presents a broad differential diagnosis to the clinician. Those with signs of severe poisoning such as altered level of consciousness, seizures, hypotension, and acidosis could have been exposed to a large number of toxicants such as salicylates, tricyclic antidepressants, isoniazid, strychnine, toxic alcohols, organic phosphorous compounds, methemoglobin-producing agents, and others. A history of gas exposure or sudden collapse of multiple victims narrows the differential to include hydrogen sulfide, carbon monoxide, azides, asphyxiants (eg, carbon dioxide, methane), phosphine, methyl halides, and arsine [4,7]. Nerve agents such as sarin can also cause rapid loss of consciousness and seizures, but the clinical effects of cholinesterase inhibition (ie, cholinergic syndrome with bradycardia, hypotension, bronchospasm, diaphoresis, nausea/vomiting, and diarrhea) should also be present. The effects of low doses of cyanogen chloride resemble those of any substances with irritant effects, including chlorine, chloramines, hydrogen chloride, hydrogen fluoride, ammonia, and riot control agents.

The number of potential critical care patients after a cyanide attack is difficult to estimate. Given its physical characteristics, it is difficult to generate large numbers of critical casualties with an HCN or cyanogen chloride release. Patients who do not rapidly lose consciousness will likely be able to remove themselves from the source of exposure, which effectively limits their illness. Those with large exposures that cause unconsciousness at the outset are unlikely to survive to hospital admission. Alternate attack scenarios such as poisoning food or water sources with a cyanide salt would also be unlikely to generate large numbers of patients. However, even a small number of seriously poisoned but salvageable patients could quickly overload emergency and critical care services, as these patients will require aggressive intervention and significant resources.

Decontamination

Exposures to gaseous cyanide and cyanogen chloride do not require any special decontamination efforts. After the patient is removed from the source of exposure, clothing should be removed. Greater care is required for patients exposed to a liquid or solid cyanide compound. Dermal exposures require clothing removal and washing of the skin with soap and water. Wounds should be cleansed thoroughly, as any remaining cyanide will be readily absorbed through damaged skin. If cyanide has been ingested, gastrointestinal decontamination via orogastric lavage and activated charcoal administration could limit the amount of cyanide absorbed. Activated charcoal adsorbs relatively small amounts of cyanide, but given the low lethal dose of cyanide, even small reductions in the absorbed dose could be clinically important [13,22].

Diagnostic studies

Specific testing for cyanide is not readily available to aid in the acute management of patients, but a number of routine tests can help to support the diagnosis. The two most important and universal laboratory findings after significant cyanide intoxication are an elevated plasma lactate concentration and an anion gap metabolic acidosis. As previously mentioned, cyanide inhibits oxidative phosphorylation, resulting in an excess of hydrogen ions with resultant systemic acidosis. Reliance on anaerobic metabolism results in increased lactate production from pyruvate. A number of cyanide's clinical effects can contribute to these laboratory abnormalities, including seizures, cardiac failure, shock, and catecholamine release [23,24].

Several studies have examined the utility of the plasma lactate concentration as a marker for cyanide intoxication. Baud et al [9] found that plasma lactate concentrations correlated well with blood cyanide concentrations in residential fire victims and pure cyanide intoxications [23]. A plasma lactate concentration >8 mmol/L was found to be 94% sensitive and 70% specific in predicting a blood cyanide concentration of >1.0 mg/L in the latter study. The negative predictive value was 98%. Exclusion of patients who had been treated with catecholamines increased the specificity, presumably due to catecholamines' effect of increasing lactate production. The investigators stress that these numbers apply only to patients in whom the diagnosis of cyanide intoxication is strongly suspected. Plasma lactate concentrations are elevated in a multitude of disease processes and poisonings, serving as a nonspecific marker for critical illness. Thus, a rapidly obtainable lactate assay can be a useful screening tool only in patients with a known or suspected cyanide exposure. In this patient population, a relatively normal plasma lactate concentration strongly argues against significant cyanide poisoning, while a significantly elevated concentration suggests the need for an antidote. Measurements of serial lactate concentrations can aid in assessing the response to antidotal therapy and need for repeat dosing [23].

Specific testing for cyanide can be helpful in confirming the diagnosis, although results will likely be obtained long after the definitive treatment of the patient has occurred. Unfortunately, accurate testing for cyanide is also challenging. It is difficult to measure cyanide in urine, although its metabolite, thiocyanate, can be used as a urinary marker for exposure [13]. Cyanide concentrates in red blood cells, making the whole blood cyanide concentration the most commonly used assay. However, cyanide is unstable in stored blood, so testing must be performed rapidly after sampling, and proper storage conditions must be maintained. In addition, acidification of whole blood during testing generates HCN, an effect that can falsely elevate the result [4]. Postmortem tissue cyanide concentrations measured in organs such as the liver and heart may be more accurate. Blood cyanide concentrations do correlate with severity of poisoning. Signs and symptoms such as flushing and tachycardia occur at 0.5 to 1.0 mg/L, obtundation at 1.0 to 2.5 mg/L, coma at 2.5 to 3.0 mg/L, and death at 3.0 mg/L [1].

Other diagnostic testing can aid in making the diagnosis of cyanide intoxication. Arterial blood sent for analysis by co-oximetry provides a number of useful pieces of information. In addition to pH and pO2, measurements of carboxyhemoglobin and methemoglobin concentrations help to rule out carbon monoxide and methemoglobin-producing agents, which can give a similar clinical picture. An elevated mixed venous oxygen saturation, measured from a central venous or pulmonary artery catheter, is an indicator of the decreased oxygen use that occurs with cyanide. This finding can also be the result of other poisons that target oxidative phosphorylation, such as carbon monoxide, sodium azide, and hydrogen sulfide [4]. Other nonspecific laboratory abnormalities include an elevated glucose concentration [23]. A study examining electrocardiograms of prisoners executed by HCN inhalation found a gradual shortening of ST segments resulting in T-wave origination on the R wave [25].

Antidotes

The goals of antidotal therapy for cyanide poisoning are twofold: to sequester cyanide from the sites of its toxic effects, and to hasten its conversion to nontoxic metabolites. In the United States, the cyanide antidote kit is currently the treatment of choice for cyanide poisoning (Fig. 2). The kit has been previously known as the Lily or Pasadena kit, and now the Taylor Cyanide Antidote Package (Taylor Pharmaceuticals, Inc., Decatur, Illinois, a subsidiary of Akorn, Inc.), as the manufacturer has changed several times over recent years. The current Taylor kit contains three medications: amyl nitrite, sodium nitrite, and sodium thiosulfate (Table 1). The antidotal effect of nitrites for cyanide poisoning has been recognized since the late nineteenth century [26]. Nitrites are oxidizers, and act primarily by inducing the formation of methemoglobin. In this process, the ferrous (+2) iron atom in hemoglobin is converted to its ferric (+3) form. This abnormal hemoglobin cannot carry oxygen, but it does have a high affinity for

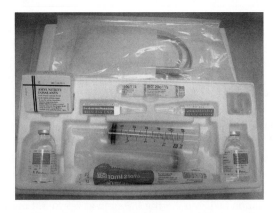

Fig. 2. Cyanide antidote kit (Taylor Pharmaceuticals, Inc., Decatur, IL, a subsidiary of Akorn, Inc.).

Table 1
Cyanide antidotes

Antidote	Mechanism of action	Side effects
Nitrites (amyl nitrite and sodium nitrite)	methemoglobin formation, ? vasodilation	reduced oxygen-carrying capacity of blood, hypotension
Sodium thiosulfate	substrate for cyanide metabolism	none significant
Hydroxocobalamin	directly binds cyanide	hypertension, transient discoloration of secretions
4-Dimethylaminophenol	methemoglobin formation	reduced oxygen-carrying capacity of blood, necrosis at injection site
Dicobalt edetate	directly binds cyanide	cardiovascular toxicity and angioedema

cyanide, even higher than that of the ferric iron in cytochrome a_3. Thus, methemoglobin can bind and sequester some of the body burden of cyanide in the blood as cyanomethemoglobin, keeping the poison away from mitochondrial and other enzymes where it exerts its toxic effects [1,27]. Interestingly, there is some data suggesting other mechanisms for the antidotal effect of nitrites. In addition to inducing methemoglobin formation, nitrites act as potent vasodilators by releasing nitric oxide. This vasodilation has been suggested to increase cyanide metabolism by increasing blood flow to the liver and other sites of detoxification [28,29]. Other vasodilators, such as chlorpromazine and phenoxybenzamine, neither of which induce methemoglobin formation, have also been found to have protective effects against cyanide toxicity [30,31].

In addition to the nitrites, sodium thiosulfate is routinely administered as a cyanide antidote, acting as a substrate for cyanide detoxification reactions. The primary pathway of cyanide metabolism is combination with sulfane sulfur to form thiocyanate (SCN−), which is far less toxic and excreted in the urine. The mitochondrial enzyme rhodanese is considered a key contributor to this process. Other important sulfurtransferases involved in thiocyanate production include 3-mercaptopyruvate sulfurtransferase and thiosulfate reductase [1]. Another important contributor may be sulfane–albumin complexes in the blood, which combine nonenzymatically with cyanide to form thiocyanate. When a significant dose of cyanide enters the body, the supply of endogenous sulfur donors is quickly exhausted by these processes. Administration of thiosulfate provides an additional sulfur source and facilitates continued cyanide metabolism [4].

Nitrites and thiosulfate are administered in combination due to their differing but synergistic effects in antagonizing cyanide. In one animal model, the lethal dose of cyanide was increased threefold after nitrite administration and fourfold after thiosulfate. Combining the two antidotes increased the lethal dose by 13 times [32]. For this reason, the combined nitrite/thiosulfate antidote regimen was introduced in the 1930s. In the current Taylor kit, amyl nitrite is supplied as a 12 separate 0.3-mL breakable glass ampules or "pearls." Two sodium nitrite 10-mL ampules each containing 300 mg in solution and two 12.5 g sodium thiosulfate bottles in 50 mL solution are included. The kit contains instructions and supplies for administering the medications, including two syringes, a 20-gauge needle, and tourniquet. Also included are a nasogastric tube and 60-mL syringe intended for use in gastric lavage. The average wholesale cost for a kit is about $200. The amyl nitrite is intended to be given before intravenous access to rapidly begin the production of methemoglobin. The package insert recommends breaking ampules one at a time in a handkerchief, which is then held in front of the patient's mouth 15 seconds at a time, followed by 15 seconds off. This process is to be repeated until the intravenous sodium nitrite can be administered. Various techniques have been recommended for amyl nitrite delivery to patients undergoing assisted ventilation. The broken ampule is simply held in front of the intake valve of a bag-valve ventilation system. Alternately, the ampule is placed in an aerosol chamber in line with airflow from a bag-valve ventilation system or ventilator, with a separate flow of oxygen flowing through the chamber [28]. If intravenous access can be readily obtained, the amyl nitrite need not be used, as sodium nitrite can be infused. A dose of 300 mg (one 10 mL ampule) should be infused over 2 to 4 minutes. Dosing for children is 6 to 8 mL/square meter of body surface area. A 12.5 g (one 50 mL bottle) dose of sodium thiosulfate should then be administered.

Unfortunately, the cyanide antidote kit, specifically the nitrite portions, can cause significant toxicity; thus, care must be taken in choosing when and how to use its contents. Nitrites can cause significant hypotension and orthostasis, so blood pressure should be carefully monitored during administration. Another significant problem is the potential for excessive production of methemoglobin, which lowers the oxygen-carrying capacity of blood to dangerous levels. This could result in low oxygen delivery to tissues in addition to the cyanide-induced impairment of aerobic energy production. Methemoglobin concentrations of less than 30% are well tolerated by otherwise healthy individuals, but concentrations of 50% to 70% or more cause serious symptoms or death. Generally, the doses of nitrite used in the antidote kit do not induce a dangerous methemoglobinemia [28]. One study of healthy subjects found a peak methemoglobin concentration of 7% after a 4 mg/kg sodium nitrite dose [33]. Another small study involving fire victims found peak concentrations of 7.9% to 13.4%, with three of four patients receiving a single 300 mg dose [34]. Nevertheless, one case report described a cyanide overdose patient who developed a methemoglobin concentration of 58% after two 300 mg sodium nitrite doses [35]. Victims of fire are at particular risk, as their oxygen-carrying capacity is already reduced by carbon monoxide exposure and formation of carboxyhemoglobin. Special care is also needed with the anemic and children, as nitrite forms methemoglobin on an equimolar basis, causing a proportionally larger amount of methemoglobin formation for a given dose. One pediatric fatality attributed to nitrite therapy for a nontoxic cyanide exposure has been reported [36]. Thus, the dosage of sodium nitrite should be carefully calculated for pediatric patients. In addition, obtain a rapid bedside measurement of hemoglobin concentration (as can be performed by many blood gas analyzers) if possible to guide dosing [28]. In contrast to the nitrites, thiosulfate has little potential for toxicity.

Given the potential complications, several limitations should be placed on use of the cyanide antidote kit. Patients in whom the diagnosis of significant cyanide poisoning is highly likely should be treated with both nitrite and thiosulfate. In cases of lower clinical suspicion, or where significant signs and symptoms are not present, the nitrite should be withheld. In fire victims, thiosulfate alone should be probably be given initially, with nitrite reserved for refractory cases or in patients in whom a rapid determination of carboxyhemoglobin concentration is obtained [28]. It should be noted, however, that in one small study of fire victims peak carboxyhemoglobin concentrations fell rapidly upon 100% oxygen therapy (mean half-life of 51 minutes) while peak methemoglobin concentrations were not achieved for 35 to 70 minutes after nitrite administration [34]. Therefore, carboxyhemoglobin concentration will likely be falling to much safer levels as the peak methemoglobin concentration is reached.

Another drug, used as a cyanide antidote in France but not currently in the United States, is hydroxocobalamin (vitamin B_{12a}) (see Table 1). It is a precursor of cyanocobalamin (vitamin B_{12}), and is used as a vitamin supplement and for the treatment of pernicious anemia. Hydroxocobalamin contains a cobalt moiety that avidly binds cyanide to form nontoxic cyanocobalamin, which is then eliminated in the urine. The drug has several properties that make it a superior antidote [6]. Hydroxocobalamin has been shown to bind cyanide intracellularly, unlike the nitrite-generated methemoglobin that is sequestered in the blood [37]. Hydroxo-cobalamin also lacks the serious potential side effects of the nitrites, making it more useful for patients such as fire victims in whom methemoglobin formation could be dangerous. The most common reaction is a reddish discoloration of the urine, skin, and mucous membranes that resolves in 1 to 2 days. A transient increase in blood pressure can also occur. A group of healthy volunteers was found to have mean increase of 13.6% in systolic and 25.9% in diastolic blood pressure after a 5 g hydroxocobalamin infusion [38]. At therapeutic doses, the intense red color of the drug also causes interfere with several common color-imetric laboratory tests, including magnesium, creatinine, bilirubin, and aspartate aminotransferase [39]. Anaphylactic reactions to hydroxocobalamin have been reported, but only after chronic use [6].

Hydroxocobalamin, packaged as the Cyanokit (Orphan Europe SARL, Paris, France), was approved in France in 1996. It is now routinely used for cyanide intoxication and is often administered to smoke inhalation victims in the prehospital setting [6]. The drug is administered in a 5 g dose over 20 to 30 minutes, which can be repeated if needed. The pediatric dose is 70 mg/kg. Sodium thiosulfate is routinely administered along with the hydroxocobalamin. Currently, the United States Food and Drug Administration (FDA) approved hydroxocobalamin formulation is too dilute for practical use as an antidote, as a 5 g dose would require a 5 L volume of the drug solution [6]. A United States version of the Cyanokit is currently in the FDA approval process, and could be available in 2006.

Other cyanide antidotes have been proposed or are in use in other countries. Alternate methemoglobin inducing drugs include 4-dimethylaminophenol, which is in use in Germany (see Table 1). Peak methemoglobin concentration occurs in 5 minutes, significantly sooner than sodium nitrite's peak effect [13]. Another advantage is its suitability for intramuscular administration, although side effects include pain and necrosis at the injection site and fever. The drug can also cause excessive methemoglobin concentrations. Another cobalt agent, dicobalt edetate (Kelocyanor), is used in the United Kingdom (see Table 1). This drug is an effective cyanide chelator, but can cause serious cardiovascular toxicity and angioedema [1]. Other experimental antidotes include stroma-free methemoglobin, α-ketoglutarate, dihydroxyacetone, and nitric oxide [3,4].

One final antidote of note is oxygen. Ventilation with 100% oxygen is an important aspect of the initial supportive care of the cyanide-intoxicated patient. In addition to helping maintain adequate tissue oxygenation, this therapy may have some synergistic effect with other antidotes. Oxygen may help displace cyanide from the cytochrome enzyme and increase the detoxification and elimination of the poison [3].

Hyperbaric oxygen therapy has been used in conjunction with antidotal therapies in a number of cyanide poisoning cases [40,41]. However, hyperbaric oxygen is currently only recommended when a concurrent carbon monoxide poisoning has occurred [42].

Supportive care

Aggressive supportive care is critical to successful antidote use and survival in the cyanide-intoxicated patient. The goals of care in the early stages of poisoning are to maintain adequate tissue perfusion and oxygenation while antidotal treatment and endogenous mechanisms reduce the availability of free cyanide at the sites of its toxic effects. Basic interventions such as high flow oxygen, large-bore intravenous lines, and cardiac monitoring are essential. As mentioned previously, supplemental oxygen may have antidotal effects in addition to its usual benefit in patients with respiratory compromise and critical illness. Endotracheal intubation for airway protection and mechanical ventilation is often necessary for the seriously poisoned patient, where vomiting, seizures, and altered level consciousness create a risk of aspiration and hypoxia. Cardiopulmonary resuscitation with concurrent administration of advanced cardiac life support medications and antidotes can also be necessary in the early stages of treatment. Intravenous crystalloids and vasopressors are useful for the hypotension that results from both the cyanide toxicity and nitrite therapy. Seizures should be treated with benzodiazepines. Intravenous sodium bicarbonate aids in the correction of the metabolic acidosis that is present in any significant cyanide intoxication. Patients with significant dermal aqueous cyanide exposure and fire victims often require extensive burn care including aggressive fluid maintenance therapy. Hemodialysis has also been advocated as a useful therapy for cyanide intoxication. Potential benefits include improvement of acidosis and increased clearance of both cyanide and its metabolite thiocyanate, particularly in the circumstance of acute or chronic renal insufficiency [43].

Clinical course and prognostic factors

The clinical course and prognosis after cyanide intoxication depend on several factors, including the type of cyanide compound involved, dose, premorbid condition of the patient, presence of concurrent poisoning or trauma, and availability of antidotal therapy. Patients who are able to remove themselves from a gaseous HCN exposure can be expected to recover quickly with little or no treatment. Oral or large dermal exposures present the problem of ongoing cyanide absorption even after medical care has been initiated. Even in this group, patients who present with coma and other signs of severe toxicity can fully recover within hours after aggressive treatment. For example, Mannaioni et al [44] reported the case of an 80-year-old man who presented comatose after ingesting a potassium cyanide solution. The patient had an initial blood pressure of 90/60 mmHg, arterial pH of 7.15, and lactate concentration of 9.2 mmol/L. After treatment including mechanical ventilation, antidotes, and sodium bicarbonate, the patient awoke with normal neurologic function within 12 hours. In contrast, another report described the suicide of an 83-year-old man, who, unlike the previous case, presented after resuscitation from a brief period of pulseless electrical activity in the field. He was hypotensive, comatose, and initial laboratory tests revealed a pH of 7.1 and lactate concentration of 6.3 mmol/L. His hemodynamics stabilized with supportive care, and several hours later, a history of cyanide ingestion was obtained. Antidotal therapy was then initiated, but the patient made no neurologic recovery and was later pronounced brain dead [45]. It is important to note that in such cases cyanide poisoning does not preclude the use of organs, including heart, liver, and kidneys, for transplantation [46].

Two important cyanide effects that can complicate the clinical course include lung and central nervous system injury. Cyanogen chloride causes a delayed pulmonary toxicity similar to phosgene. Lung injury, with pulmonary edema and adult respiratory distress syndrome, can occur in the clinical course of any serious cyanide overdose [13]. Brain injury similar to that after exposure to other toxicants such as carbon monoxide and hydrogen sulfide has also been reported. The pattern of central nervous system injury ranges from brain death to subtle injuries to the most sensitive areas such as the basal ganglia. Patients can develop delayed neurologic sequellae, manifesting days to months after the initial poisoning. Parkinsonian symptoms occur before or concurrently with dystonia. Symptoms include bradykinesia, dysarthria, rigidity, and ataxia. Neuroimaging most often reveals injury to the putamen and globus pallidus, while the cerebral cortex, cerebellum, and other areas can also show abnormalities [47,48]. Treatment with dopaminergic agents has yielded significant clinical improvement in some patients but is often of no benefit [49].

References

[1] Baskin SI, Brewer TG. Cyanide poisoning. In: Sidell FR, Takefuji ET, Franz DR, editors. Medical aspects of chemical and biological warfare. Washington, DC: Office of the Surgeon General; 1997. p. 271–86.

[2] Cummings TF. The treatment of cyanide poisoning. Occup Med (Lond) 2004;54(2):82–5.

[3] Gracia R, Shepherd G. Cyanide poisoning and its treatment. Pharmacotherapy 2004;24(10): 1358–65.

[4] Curry SC, LoVecchio FA. Hydrogen cyanide and inorganic cyanide salts. In: Sullivan JB, Krieger GR, editors. Clinical environmental health and toxic exposures. 2nd edition. Philadelphia: Lippincott Williams & Wilkins; 2001. p. 705–16.

[5] Pennardt A. CBRNE—cyanides, hydrogen. www.emedicine.com/emerg/topic909.htm. Accessed March 30, 2004.

[6] Sauer SW, Keim ME. Hydroxocobalamin: improved public health readiness for cyanide disasters. Ann Emerg Med 2001;37(6):635–41.

[7] Eckstein M. Cyanide as a chemical terrorism weapon. JEMS 2004;29(8; Suppl):22–31.

[8] Alcorta R. Smoke inhalation and acute cyanide poisoning. JEMS 2004;29(8, Suppl):6–15.

[9] Baud FJ, Barriot P, Toffis V, et al. Elevated blood cyanide concentrations in victims of smoke inhalation. N Engl J Med 1991;325(25):1761–6.

[10] Silverman SH, Purdue GF, Hunt JL, et al. Cyanide toxicity in burned patients. J Trauma 1988; 28(2):171–6.

[11] Yeoh MJ, Braitberg G. Carbon monoxide and cyanide poisoning in fire related deaths in Victoria, Australia. J Toxicol Clin Toxicol 2004;42(6):855–63.

[12] Martinez JA. CBRNE—cyanides, cyanogen chloride. www.emedicine.com/emerg/topic910.htm. Accessed March 30, 2004.

[13] Kerns W, Isom G, Kirk MA. Cyanide and hydrogen sulfide. In: Goldfrank LR, Flomenbaum NE, Lewin NA, Howland MA, Hoffman RS, Nelson LS, editors. Goldfrank's toxicologic emergencies. 7th edition. New York: McGraw-Hill; 2002. p. 1498–510.

[14] Mizock BA. Controversies in lactic acidosis. JAMA 1987;258(4):497–501.

[15] Ballantyne B. An experimental assessment of the diagnostic potential of histochemical and biochemical methods for cytochrome oxidase in acute cyanide poisoning. Cell Mol Biol Incl Cyto Enzymol 1977;22(1):109–23.

[16] Ardelt BK, Borowitz JL, Isom GE. Brain lipid peroxidation and antioxidant protectant mechanisms following acute cyanide intoxication. Toxicology 1989;56(2):147–54.

[17] Patel MN, Yim GK, Isom GE. N-methyl-D-aspartate receptors mediate cyanide-induced cytotoxicity in hippocampal cultures. Neurotoxicology 1993;14(1):35–40.

[18] Rosenow F, Herholz K, Lanfermann H, et al. Neurological sequelae of cyanide intoxication—the patterns of clinical, magnetic resonance imaging, and positron emission tomography findings. Ann Neurol 1995;38(5):825–8.

[19] Tursky T, Sajter V. The influence of potassium cyanide poisoning on the gamma-aminobutyric acid level in rat brain. J Neurochem 1962;9:519–23.

[20] Gonzalez ER. Cyanide evades some noses, overpowers others. JAMA 1982;248(18):2211.

[21] Johnson RP, Mellors JW. Arteriolization of venous blood gases: a clue to the diagnosis of cyanide poisoning. J Emerg Med 1988;6(5):401–4.

[22] Lambert RJ, Kindler BL, Schaeffer DJ. The efficacy of superactivated charcoal in treating rats exposed to a lethal oral dose of potassium cyanide. Ann Emerg Med 1988;17(6): 595–8.

[23] Baud FJ, Borron SW, Megarbane B, et al. Value of lactic acidosis in the assessment of the severity of acute cyanide poisoning. Crit Care Med 2002;30(9):2044–50.

[24] Kanthasamy AG, Borowitz JL, Isom GE. Cyanide-induced increases in plasma catecholamines: relationship to acute toxicity. Neurotoxicology 1991;12(4):777–84.

[25] Wexler J, Whittenberger JL, Dumke PR. The effect of cyanide on the electrocardiogram of man. Am Heart J 1947;34:163–73.

[26] Pedigo LG. Antagonism between amyl nitrite and prussic acid. Trans Med Soc Virginia 1888; 19:124–31.

[27] Smith L, Kruszyna H, Smith RP. The effect of methemoglobin on the inhibition of cytochrome c oxidase by cyanide, sulfide or azide. Biochem Pharmacol 1977;26(23):2247–50.

[28] Kerns W. Cyanide antidotes. In: Goldfrank LR, Flomenbaum NE, Lewin NA, Howland MA, Hoffman RS, Nelson LS, editors. Goldfrank's toxicologic emergencies. 7th edition. New York: McGraw-Hill; 2002. p. 1511–4.

[29] Tamulinas CB, Nizamani S, Myers M. The effect of blood flow on cyanide metabolism in the isolated perfused rat liver. Fed Proc 1985;44:1796.

[30] Gurrows GE, Way JL. Antagonism of cyanide toxicity by phenoxybenzamine. Fed Proc 1975;36:534.

[31] Pettersen JC, Cohen SD. Antagonism of cyanide poisoning by chlorpromazine and sodium thiosulfate. Toxicol Appl Pharmacol 1985;81(2):265–73.

[32] Chen KK, Rose RL, Clowes GHA. Methylene blue, nitrites, and sodium thiosulphate against cyanide poisoning. Proc Soc Exp Biol Med 1933;31:250–1.

[33] Kiese M, Weger NP. Formation of ferrihemoglobin with the aminophenols in the human for the treatment of cyanide poisoning. Eur J Pharmacol 1969;7(1):97–105.

[34] Kirk MA, Gerace R, Kulig KW. Cyanide and methemoglobin kinetics in smoke inhalation victims treated with the cyanide antidote kit. Ann Emerg Med 1993;22(9):1413–8.

[35] van Heijst AN, Douze JM, van Kesteren RG, et al. Therapeutic problems in cyanide poisoning. J Toxicol Clin Toxicol 1987;25(5):383–98.

[36] Berlin CM. The treatment of cyanide poisoning in children. Pediatrics 1970;46(5):793–6.

[37] Astier A, Baud FJ. Simultaneous determination of hydroxocobalamin and its cyanide complex cyanocobalamin in human plasma by high-performance liquid chromatography. Application to pharmacokinetic studies after high-dose hydroxocobalamin as an antidote for severe cyanide poisoning. Chromatogr B Biomed Appl 1995;667(1):129–35.

[38] Forsyth JC, Mueller PD, Becker CE, et al. Hydroxocobalamin as a cyanide antidote: safety, efficacy, and pharmacokinetics in heavily smoking normal volunteers. J Toxicol Clin Toxicol 1993;31(2):277–94.

[39] Curry SC, Connor DA, Raschke RA. Effect of the cyanide antidote hydroxocobalamin on commonly ordered serum chemistry studies. Ann Emerg Med 1994;24(1):65–7.

[40] Litovitz TL, Larkin RF, Myers RA. Cyanide poisoning treated with hyperbaric oxygen. Am J Emerg Med 1983;1(1):94–101.

[41] Goodhart GL. Patient treated with antidote kit and hyperbaric oxygen survives cyanide poisoning. South Med J 1994;87(8):814–6.

[42] Weiss LD, Van Meter KW. The applications of hyperbaric oxygen therapy in emergency medicine. Am J Emerg Med 1992;10(6):558–68.

[43] Wesson DE, Foley R, Sabatini S, et al. Treatment of acute cyanide intoxication with hemodialysis. Am J Nephrol 1985;5(2):121–6.

[44] Mannaioni G, Vannacci A, Marzocca C, et al. Acute cyanide intoxication treated with a combination of hydroxycobalamin, sodium nitrite, and sodium thiosulfate. J Toxicol Clin Toxicol 2002;40(2):181–3.

[45] Mutlu GM, Leiken JB, Oh K, et al. An unresponsive biochemistry professor in the bathtub. Chest 2002;122(3):1073–6.

[46] Swanson-Biearman B, Krenzelok EP, Snyder JW, et al. Successful donation and transplantation of multiple organs from a victim of cyanide poisoning. J Toxicol Clin Toxicol 1993;31(1):95–9.

[47] Martin CO, Adams HP. Neurological aspects of biological and chemical terrorism. Arch Neurol 2003;60(1):21–5.

[48] Albin RL. Basal ganglia neurotoxins. Neurol Clin 2000;18(3):665–80.

[49] Borgohain R, Singh AK, Radhakrishna H, Mohanda S. Delayed onset generalized dystonia after cyanide poisoning. Clin Neurol Neurosurg 1995;97(3):213–5.

ELSEVIER
SAUNDERS

CRITICAL
CARE
CLINICS

Crit Care Clin 21 (2005) 707–718

Vesicants

John McManus, MD, MCR, FACEP[a],*, Kermit Huebner, MD[b]

[a]US Army Institute of Surgical Research, 3400 Rawley E. Chambers Avenue,
Fort Sam Houston, TX 78234-6315, USA
[b]US Army Medical Research Institute of Infectious Diseases, 1425 Porter Street,
Fort Detrick, MD 21702, USA

Gas! GAS! Quick, boys!
An ecstasy of fumbling
Fitting the clumsy helmets just in time,
But someone still was
yelling out and stumbling
And flound'ring like a man in fire or lime–
Dim through the misty panes
and thick green light,
As under a green sea, I saw him drowning.
In all my dreams before my helpless sight
He plunges at me, guttering, choking, drowning.

(British poet Wilfried Owen, 1918)

From the use of smoke by the Mohist sect in China in fourth century BC through the use of incendiary shells filled with sulfa and belladonna in the fifteenth century, the use of chemicals and irritants during battle has been well documented throughout the centuries. However, most sources credit the origin of modern chemical warfare to the German's release of thousands of cylinders of chlorine gas on French and Algerian troops near Ypres, Belgium, in April of 1915 during World War I (WWI) [1]. Use of chemicals had already escalated

---

The opinions or assertions expressed herein are the private views of the authors and are not to be construed as official or as reflecting the views of the US Department of the Army or the US Department of Defense.

The pulmonary aspects of blistering agents overlap the material on irritant gases in the respiratory agents article. We have kept these articles and inclusive topics as separate discussions with unique and complementary features.

* Corresponding author.
E-mail address: john.mcmanus@amedd.army.mil (J. McManus).

during the previous year by the French who used chloroacetone, and by the Germans who used odianisidine chlorosulfonate. These chemical weapons reduced combat effectiveness of enemy forces through logistical disruption and by inflicting injury rather than by causing direct mortality. Approximately 125,000 tons of chemical agents were used during WWI and produced an estimated 1.3 million casualties [2]. The use of vesicants, particularly sulfur mustard, was responsible for nearly 80% of the casualties and sulfur mustard became known as "king of the battle gases" [1].

Vesicants (blister agents) are cytotoxic alkylating compounds that are chemical agents sometimes collectively known as "mustard gas" or simply "mustard" (military designator: H). Other blister agents are nitrogen mustard (HN); sulfur mustard (HD); lewisite (L), a vesicant that contains arsenic; and phosgene oxime (CX), a halogenated oxime that has different properties and toxicity from the other agents. Blister agents are an exception to the limited utility of classic chemical agents. These agents have been used effectively and extensively throughout modern warfare. Vesicants are rarely lethal but they inflict painful burns and blisters, which require medical attention even at low doses. Because vesicants can inflict many casualties and create confusion and panic, they were used in battle throughout the twentieth century.

The 1925 Geneva Protocol [3], which was endorsed by many world nations, included a pledge to never use gas or bacteriologic methods of warfare; however, chemical agents, specifically mustard, have been used continually since WWI. Italy allegedly used mustard in the 1930s against Abyssinia during the invasion of Ethiopia. The Japanese used both mustard and lewisite agents against Chinese troops from 1937 to 1944. Although Egypt denies allegations, they were accused of using mustard and nerve agents in the 1960s against Yemen [3]. Most recently, Iraq used mustard against Iran and against the Kurds during the 1980s. As many as 34,000 Iranians were known to have been exposed to sulfur mustard, which resulted in many chronic medical problems [4].

Mechanism of toxicity

Proposed use as a weapon

Exposure to vesicants may occur in a variety of settings. Environmental exposures are possible in areas where chemical weapons are produced, tested, or stored. Additionally, the Environmental Protection Agency has located sites where sulfur mustard can be found in contaminated soil or containers [5]. Sulfur mustard may also be found at sea. Dumping sulfur mustard at sea was a standard method of disposal from WWI until the 1970s, and accounts of sulfur mustard surfacing during fishing expeditions have been reported. Stockpiles of chemical munitions still exist in the United States; however, according to the international Chemical Weapons treaty, these stockpiles of mustard agents must be destroyed by April 2007. The most likely exposure scenario is occupational exposure, caused by aged storage containers, of personnel working with these agents in storage facilities or depots. A 100-gallon spill from a 1-ton container occurred in 1993 at Tooele Army Depot, Utah, and other leaking munitions have been discovered as recently as 2002 [5].

The greatest concern today is the use of a vesicant agent in a terrorist attack. Unlike environmental or occupational exposures, the use of a vesicant agent by a terrorist has the potential to create a significant number of casualties. Additionally, the use of these agents has the potential to (1) create fear and panic because of the grotesque nature of the injuries inflicted, (2) overwhelm the medical infrastructure, and (3) substantially impact the nation's economy. The factor that limits terrorist use is acquisition of the vesicant agent. Fortunately, security at United States military storage sites is significant; however, there are several other countries that are known to have chemical munitions, including vesicants, or possess the knowledge to produce these weapons [3].

Method of exposure

Vesicants burn and blister any part of the body they contact. They act on the eyes, mucous membranes, lungs, skin, and blood-forming organs. They damage the respiratory tract when inhaled, and cause vomiting and diarrhea when ingested. The vesicant agents may be released in several ways, depending on the agent and its physical characteristics. Sulfur mustard is an oily liquid with low volatility and a freezing point of 58°F (14°C) [6]. Lewisite is also an oily liquid that is more volatile than sulfur mustard and has a freezing point of 0.4°F (−18°C) [7]. Phosgene oxime is a solid in the pure form, but munitions grade phosgene oxime is a yellowish brown liquid with a melting point of 95°F to 104°F (35°C to 40°C) [8]. Exposures may include skin contact (even through clothing), inhalation of vapors, and ingestion of the chemical.

The most damaging method of exposure is inhalation of the chemical agent. The physical properties of sulfur mustard make it a better weapon for use in warm environments, where there is greater risk of vapor inhalation; lewisite is a better weapon in colder environments because of its increased volatility. Lewisite may be mixed with sulfur mustard to lower the freezing point of sulfur mustard and increase its effectiveness at lower temperatures [3]. Once it is released into the environment, these compounds may persist for up to a week in temperate climates. Furthermore, vesicant agents can be thickened to contaminate terrain, ships, aircraft, vehicles, or equipment with a persistent hazard.

Biochemical, cellular, and systemic effects

Although chemical agents have been studied, produced, and developed as weapons by several countries, the exact mechanism of action of vesicant agents remains unknown. Sulfur mustard exerts it effects on the cellular level by acting as an electrophile that combines with macromolecules in the cell, including proteins, RNA, DNA, and components of the cell membrane. The end result of these interactions is cell death— either by necrosis, apoptosis, or a combination of both. Theories about the cause of cell death have focused on the alkylation of DNA and reactions with glutathione. The initial step in the cytotoxic pathway may be irreversible alkylation of purines in DNA, which leads to random nuclear DNA fragmentation. The DNA damage activates a polymerase enzyme that depletes NAD and inhibits synthesis of ATP, which leads to cell death [9]. Pretreating cells with N-acetylcysteine has shown benefits in some studies; therefore, it is theorized that cell apoptosis after exposure to sulfur mustard may be related to depletion of reduced glutathione, which results in an increase in free radicals and leads to lipid peroxidation. Cellular death and interactions with cytoskeletal organization leads to decreased cellular adherence and morphologic changes in tissues. Evaluation of endothelial cells revealed that rounding of adherent cells and changes in polymerized actin were visible as early as 2 hours after exposure to sulfur mustard [10].

Histopathological changes in an animal model have demonstrated individual cell death within 2 hours of vapor exposure, and generalized necrosis beginning within 12 hours after exposure. Basement membrane degeneration follows and leads to microblisters, which coalesce to form larger blisters in human exposure. Damage to the upper dermis appears to be an inflammatory response with vascular endothelial swelling and vacuolization, dermal edema, and inflammatory cell infiltrates [11].

Lewisite is arsenic, not an alkylating agent. Arsenics are reported to inhibit the activity of enzymes that contain adjacent sulfhydryl groups, which leads to NADPH and glutathione oxidation. Therefore, membrane damage and disruption of cell metabolism leads to cell death, necrosis, and skin blistering [12].

The mechanism of action of phosgene oxime is unknown, but may be related to the necrotizing effects of the chlorine, the direct effect of the oxime, or the effect of its carbonyl group. The skin lesions of phosgene oxime are not blisters and, therefore, it is not a true vesicant agent. Instead of the blisters seen with sulfur mustard and lewisite, phosgene oxime lesions are wheals that may be followed by dark eschars [3].

Clinical presentation

The clinical signs and symptoms of exposure to a vesicant agent will depend on the route of administration and the vesicant agent used. The predominant organs affected are the skin, eyes, and lungs. Sulfur mustard casualties from WWI and the Iran-Iraq war manifested effects from multiple routes of exposure (cutaneous and ocular lesions from liquid mustard or mustard vapor exposure and respiratory symptoms from inhalation of mustard vapor) [5]. Systemic effects may occur and are radiomimetic in nature.

Cutaneous exposure

Skin exposure can occur from contact with the solid, liquid, or vapor form of a vesicant agent. A 10 microgram liquid droplet is enough to produce skin lesions, and vapor exposure at 200 mg/min/m^3 can produce lesions. Lesions progress from erythema, beginning within 4–8 hours after exposure, to the development of vesicles in 2–18 hours, which then coalesce to form large blisters over days. The lesions are superficial, translucent, and approximately 0.5–5.0 cm in diameter, but may vary in size. The fluid inside the blister does not contain mustard and is not an exposure threat to health care workers [3]. Mustard lesions differ from thermal burns in that they usually are partial thickness and tend to have slower spontaneous healing rates [13]. Lesions may not heal for weeks or for several months, depending on the location and depth of the injury [3].

Unlike exposure to sulfur mustard, which is painless until the development of erythema, exposure to lewisite typically produces pain and irritation within minutes of exposure. The lewisite blister develops within minutes and expands, unlike the development of multiple vesicles that merge in sulfur mustard lesions [3]. Additionally, lewisite lesions are comparable to thermal burns and heal faster than mustard lesions [13].

Phosgene oxime is not a true vesicant and does not produce blisters. Exposure to phosgene oxime leads to immediate pain, followed by a grayish skin lesion surrounded by erythema. Edema forms around the edge of the lesion and central necrosis ensues with the development of a wheal that regresses over 24 hours and is replaced with a dark eschar [3].

Ocular exposure

The eye is the most sensitive tissue to mustard vapor and can shows signs of irritation at concentrations 10 times lower than the concentration required to affect the airways [14]. In an evaluation of more than 5000 mustard casualties from the Iran-Iraq war, most had ocular symptoms and 10% developed severe ocular damage [15]. Most of the casualties suffered from conjunctivitis, eyelid edema, and blepharospasm. Conjunctival exposure leads to rapid vasodilation, increased vascular permeability, and edema. The corneal epithelium develops vesicles and begins to slough several hours later [16]. More serious symptoms included visual disturbances, keratitis, and corneal ulceration. Approximately 90% of the patients recovered, although in some patients, symptoms of conjunctivitis and photosensitivity persisted for several months [15]. Ocular exposure to lewisite also results in edema of the eyelids, conjunctiva, and cornea. With lewisite exposures, the patient suffers immediate pain and irritation that produces blepharospasm, which helps prevent further exposure [3]. Phosgene oxime causes ocular symptoms similar to lewisite with immediate pain and irritation, conjunctivitis, and keratitis.

Inhalation

Inhalation of mustard vapor leads to damage of the respiratory tree and symptoms typically develop within 4–6 hours of the exposure. Symptoms begin in the upper airways and progress to the lower airways as the dose and time of exposure are increased. Initial symptoms may include a sore throat, hoarseness, and cough which can progress to laryngospasm, bronchospasm, and severe dyspnea [17]. Blister formation and necrosis of the upper airways may lead to pseudomembrane formation and airway obstruction up to several days after the exposure. Exposures to high concentrations may produce severe symptoms more rapidly and can lead to hemorrhagic bronchitis [18]. The incidence of pulmonary infections in mustard inhalation casualties is high and was a major cause of mortality in American soldiers during WWI. Lewisite vapor exposure results in a clinical syndrome similar to that of mustard; however, the irritating effects of lewisite are manifested much sooner. Exposure to large concentrations of lewisite may result in pulmonary edema. Exposure to phosgene oxime vapor may lead to pulmonary edema, necrotizing bronchiolitis, and pulmonary venule thrombosis [18]. Initial death, although rare with vesicant exposure, is usually the result of suffocation.

Systemic effects

Sulfur mustard has a profound effect on rapidly dividing cells and is often described as a radiomimetic agent. Reports of casualties from WWI and the Iran-Iraq war reveal hematologic effects that include leukocytosis after the injury, followed by leucopenia, and sometimes pancytopenia 3–4 days after the exposure. Leukopenia may be severe: white blood cell counts ≤ 200 cells/μL. Mustard is also mutagenic and has been linked to a slight, but statistically significant incidence of lung cancer deaths in mustard casualties from WWI. A study that followed German factory workers with occupational exposures to sulfur mustard for a 20-year period, revealed a statistically significant increase in bronchial carcinoma, bladder carcinoma, and leukemia [19]. Lewisite has not been shown to affect the hematopoeitic system and has not been associated with an increase in malignant tumors. However, lewisite may cause "lewisite shock." Exposure to large amounts of lewisite may result in systemic absorption that leads to capillary damage and results in protein and plasma leakage with hemoconcentration and hypotension [3].

Differential diagnosis

The differential diagnosis for vesicant exposure can be quite large, but can be narrowed down with a comprehensive history and physical examination. The differential diagnosis may include thermal burns, other chemical burns, pemphigus vulgaris, bullous pemphigoid, toxic epidermal necrolysis, staphylococcus scalded skin syndrome, and Stevens-Johnson syndrome. Although exposure to vesicants is not typically listed high on the differential diagnosis for dermatologic conditions, ocular conditions, or respiratory symptoms, history may reveal an occupational exposure or environmental exposure from old munitions. An intentional release from terrorists will result in large numbers of casualties with similar symptoms and a common source of exposure, such as a large public gathering.

Physical examination of the skin will assist in identifying the vesicant agent used. Sulfur mustard lesions are initially painless. Mustard lesions typically become painful with the onset of erythema 4–6 hours after the exposure, and develop a string of small vesicles that coalesce to form larger blisters. Lewisite causes pain and irritation at the time of exposure and leads to a vesicle that enlarges. Phosgene oxime exposure results in immediate pain, a lesion that is initially gray and develops into a wheal, followed by necrosis and a black eschar. The tricothecene mycotoxins (T-2 mycotoxins) are biologic toxins that are dermally active and cause lesions similar to sulfur mustard. The T-2 mycotoxins are also considered radiomimetic and may result in bone marrow depletion.

Casualty and injury distribution

Multiple variables will affect the number of casualties resulting from a terrorist release of vesicant agents. Considerations include the agent, the dispersal method, the ambient conditions, and the number of people near the exposure site. More than 80% of mustard casualties are from vapor exposure. Warm, moist areas of skin, such as the armpits and groin, appear to have an increased potential for damage. Of 6980 cases of mustard burns during WWI, the location of the lesions were eyes (86%), respiratory tract (75%), scrotum (42%), face (27%), anus (24%), legs (11%), buttocks (10%), hands (4%), and feet (1.5%). The overall mortality rate was 2%–3% and most fatalities were related to pulmonary complications [20].

The presentation of mustard casualties may be delayed for several hours after exposure, especially if exposed to low doses. Casualties from lewisite and phosgene oxime are more likely to present immediately after an incident because of the immediate pain and irritation that occurs. Additionally, consideration needs to be given to those that may present for evaluation that do not have symptoms or have not had a true exposure. The recommended guidance is to plan for a ratio of 5:1 (5 unaffected casualties to one affected casualty). During the sarin release in the Tokyo subway, there were 5510 victims that sought medical care at 278 different health care facilities. Of these, 12 casualties died, 17 casualties were critically ill, 37 were seriously ill, 984 were moderately ill, and 4000 victims were not exposed to any significant amount of the chemical agent [21].

Management and evaluation

Decontamination

Decontamination is mandatory to prevent continued exposure to the agent and to protect health care workers. Vesicant agents do pose a threat to health care workers if casualties are not decontaminated or are incompletely decontaminated. Full personal protective equipment is recommended until full decontamination is accomplished. Vesicant casualties need decontamination as soon as possible to prevent further injuries. The chemical agent must be physically removed to achieve successful decontamination. Victims should remove clothing, remove any visible agent on the skin, and move to an area free of vapor hazards. Physical removal may be accomplished by several methods: wiping off the agent with dry powders (such as flour, powdered soap, or dirt), showering, washing with soap and water, washing with 0.5% hypochlorite solution, or using resin decontaminants, which are used by the military [22]. Hypochlorite solutions may be used for patients immediately after the exposure; however, if skin erythema has developed, it is preferable to use soap and water rather than hypocholorite to avoid further skin injury. A comparison of decontamination effects of hypochlorite and water in an animal model has shown that similar amounts of sulfur mustard were removed by each method [23]. Hypochlorite solutions should not be used on the eyes or mucus membranes; however, eyes should be irrigated with water or saline as there tends to be a significant number of casualties that develop ocular symptoms.

Initial decontamination should occur in the pre-hospital setting near the scene of the incident. Pre-hospital personnel need to use appropriate personnel protective equipment while performing on-scene triage and decontamination. Patients should be evaluated for effectiveness of decontamination before they are transported to health care facilities. Emergency departments should expect to receive decontaminated patients from the scene by way of Emergency Medical Services (EMS), but hospital personnel will need to verify that patients have been decontaminated appropriately before allowing patients to enter the facility. If not appropriately decontaminated, health care workers may develop symptoms from exposure to solid or liquid agents, or vapors from solid or liquid agents, on the casualties. Emergency departments must also be prepared to perform decontamination on casualties that arrive by non-EMS means. Decontamination must occur outside of the health care facility by personnel wearing appropriate personal protective equipment.

Patients that are admitted to the intensive care unit should have already undergone decontamination with verification of decontamination before admission. The chance of admitting a contaminated patient to a health care facility is miniscule [22]. The blister fluid does not contain the vesicant agent and poses no threat to health care workers. However, medical personnel should wear protective gear including breathing protection if casualties are not fully decontaminated in the field. Note that chemical (butyl rubber) gloves should be worn during decontamination because latex gloves are not adequate.

Diagnostic studies

Diagnosis of vesicant exposure, without obvious contamination, requires a high index of suspicion when eye, skin, and respiratory signs and symptoms become evident. Another clue that vesicant exposure has occurred may be the smell of onion, garlic, geraniums, or fish [24]. In general, however, there is no specific medical test to determine if there has been exposure to a vesicant agent. A nonspecific finding of leukopenia may occur 3 to 5 days post-exposure, which may indicate vesicant exposure. A metabolite of mustard, thiodiglycol, has been found in higher concentration than controls in Iranian mustard casualties [25]. With the exception of urinary arsenic excretion, no specific tests exist for lewisite. Phosgene oxime has never been used on the battlefield and no specific tests are currently diagnostic and exposure is made on clinical suspicion. Sulfur mustard, nitrogen mustard, and lewisite may be definitively detected and identified for confirmation and public health and epidemiologic purposes, by sending 25 mL of urine to a regional public health laboratory as described on the website of the Centers for Disease Control and Prevention: www.bt.cdc.gov/labissues/pdf/shipping-samples.pdf and www.bt.cdc.gov/labissues/pdf/chemspecimencollection.pdf.

Antidotes

There are no specific antidotes for mustard exposure. Decontamination within minutes of exposure is the best way to minimize tissue damage and toxic effects from vesicant exposure. The use of N-acetyl-cysteine was shown to decrease the inflammatory response in mustard exposure in an animal model [26]. Also, one animal study suggests that rapid application of providone iodine ointment within 20 minutes of exposure to mustard liquid, may protect the skin from vesication [23,27]. Barrier creams have also been proposed by the United States Army in the past to prevent dermal toxicity from vesicant exposure [28].

A British anti-lewisite agent (dimercaprol) can be used to bind the arsenic group in lewisite and may prevent or decrease both systemic and local toxicity by acting as a chelator. Dimercaprol may be given intramuscularly for systemic toxicity or topically within minutes of exposure for ocular or cutaneous treatment. Indications for dimercaprol administration include severe systemic signs (eg, pulmonary edema or significant burns) and should be given within 15 minutes of exposure. Consultation with the regional poison control center (1-800-222-1222, in the United States), if available, is recommended.

There is no antidote for phosgene oxime exposure and treatment is managed supportively and symptomatically.

Supportive care

Once patients are decontaminated, treatment consists of supportive and palliative measures. Mustard burns should be managed in a manner similar to thermal burns: analgesia, infection control, and fluid replacement. Antibiotic ointments and silver sulfadiazine creams are recommended for topical burn care [3]. Dermal hypersensitivity may respond to antihistamines or oral or systemic corticosteroids. All patients with ocular exposure should have contact lenses removed, if applicable, and be thoroughly irrigated with saline. Topical mydriatics, antibiotics, and limited steroids (12–24 hours) have been recommended [3,21]. Mild respiratory exposure may respond to antitussives, warm humidified air, and bronchodilators for wheezing or bronchospasm. Persistent symptoms may suggest bronchitis, pneumonia, or pneumonitis, and will require more aggressive therapies.

Although there is no literature available regarding ventilator management for mustard victims, some recent literature suggests decreased mortality with reduced tidal volumes in patients with acute lung injury and adult respiratory distress syndrome (ARDS) [29,30]. The largest of these studies, The National Institutes of Health ARDS Network [31], conducted a clinical trial of mechanical ventilation in ARDS patients, which compared 6 mL/kg predicted body weight tidal volume to 12 mL/kg predicted body weight in ventilated patients. The 6 mL/kg group had 31% mortality compared with 40% for the 12 mL/kg group. Despite the demonstrated reduction in mortality, low tidal ventilation has not gained universal acceptance. This ventilation approach may, however, protect the lungs from excessive stretch, resulting in improved clinical outcomes for patients with acute lung injury and acute respiratory distress syndrome. On the basis of these results, clinicians may consider using this low tidal ventilation protocol in patients with acute lung injury and the acute respiratory distress syndrome.

Clinical course and prognostic factors

Patients who have ocular or airway symptoms should be admitted to the hospital. Also, moderate to severe skin exposure requires hospitalization. Even patients with mild symptoms need to be observed for 18 to 24 hours for development of delayed symptoms [7]. A total white blood cell count of <500 indicates a poor prognosis. Exposure to mustard agents is also associated with developing chronic health problems including respiratory diseases (eg, asthma, pulmonary fibrosis, and bronchiectasis) [17,24,32], skin lesions (eg, dermal scarring) [28,33], neoplasms [24,34], and ocular problems (eg, keratitis, conjunctivitis and corneal ulcers) [32,35]. Also, blood counts, serum electrolytes, and coagulation times should be monitored for secondary effects of these agents.

Summary

Critical care providers and facilities should be prepared for the treatment and care of large amounts of casualties in the event of vesicant use. The basic principles for the management of vesicant exposure are containment, prevention of secondary contamination, rapid decontamination, and implementation of symptomatic and supportive care. The ability of care providers to recognize, respond, and appropriately treat chemical casualties will help minimize adverse outcomes.

References

[1] Haber LF. The poisonous cloud: chemical warfare in the first world war. Oxford, England: Charendon Press; 1986.

[2] Prentiss AM. Chemicals in war: a treatise on chemical warfare. New York: McGraw Hill; 1937.

[3] Sidell FR, Urbanetti JS, Smith WJ, et al. Vesicants. In: Zajtchuk R, Bellamy RF, editors. Textbook of military medicine. Part I: Medical aspects of chemical and biological warfare. Falls Church (VA): Office of the Surgeon General, Dept of the Army; 1997. p. 197–228.

[4] Khateri S, Ghanei M, Keshavarz S, et al. Incidence of lung, eye, and skin lesions as late complications in 34,000 Iranians with wartime exposure to mustard agent. J Occup Environ Med 2003;45(11):1136–43.

[5] Agency for Toxic Substances and Disease Registry (ATSDR) toxicologic profile of sulfur mustard (Update). Atlanta (GA): Department of Health and Human Services, Public Health Service; 2003.

[6] Medical management guidelines for blister agents: sulfur mustard agent H or HD & sulfur mustard agent HT. Available at: http://www.atsdr.cdc.gov/MHMI/mmg165.pdf. Accessed March 8, 2005.

[7] Medical management guidelines for blister agents: lewisite and mustard-lewisite mixture. Available at: http://www.atsdr.cdc.gov/MHMI/mmg163.pdf. Accessed March 8, 2005.

[8] Medical management guidelines for phosgene oxime. Available at: http://www.atsdr.cdc.gov/MHMI/mmg167.pdf. Accessed March 8, 2005.

[9] Meier HL, Gross CL, Papirmeister B. 2,2'-Dichlorodiethyl sulfide (sulfur mustard) decreases NAD + levels in human leukocytes. Toxicol Lett 1987;39(1):109–22.

[10] Dabrowska MI, Becks LL, Lelli Jr JL, et al. Sulfur mustard induces poptosis and necrosis in endothelial cells. Toxicol Appl Pharmacol 1996;141(2):568–83.

[11] Brown RF, Rice P. Histopathological changes in Yucatan minipig skin following challenge with sulphur mustard. A sequential study of the first 24 hours following challenge. Int J Exp Pathol 1997;78(1):9–20.

[12] Kehe K, Flohe S, Krebs G, et al. Effects of Lewisite on cell membrane integrity and energy metabolism in human keratinocytes and SCL II cells. Toxicology 2001;163(2–3):137–44.

[13] Chilcott RP, Jenner J, Hotchkiss SA, et al. In vitro skin absorption and decontamination of sulphur mustard: comparison of human and pig-ear skin. J Appl Toxicol 2001;21(4):279–83.

[14] Smith WJ, Dunn MA. Medical defense against blistering chemical warfare agents. Arch Dermatol 1991;127(8):1207–13.

[15] Safarinejad MR, Moosavi SA, Montazeri B. Ocular injuries caused by mustard gas: diagnosis, treatment, and medical defense. Mil Med 2001;166(1):67–70.

[16] Banin E, Morad Y, Berenshtein E, et al. Injury induced by chemical warfare agents: characterization and treatment of ocular tissues exposed to nitrogen mustard. Invest Ophthalmol Vis Sci 2003;44(7):2966–72.

[17] Parrish JS, Bradshaw DA. Toxic inhalational injury: gas, vapor and vesicant exposure. Respir Care Clin N Am 2004;10(1):43–58.

[18] Bogucki S, Weir S. Pulmonary manifestations of intentionally released chemical and biological agents. Clin Chest Med 2002;23(4):777–94.

[19] Weiss A, Weiss B. Carcinogenesis due to mustard gas exposure in man, important sign for therapy with alkylating agents. Dtsch Med Wochenschr 1975;100(17):919–23.

[20] Dire DJ. CBRNE-vesicants, mustard: HD, HN1–3, H. Available at: http://www.emedicine.com/emerg/topic901.htm. Accessed March 8, 2005.

[21] Guidelines for mass casualty decontamination during a terrorist chemical agent incident. Available at: http://www.au.af.mil/au/awc/awcgate/army/sbccom_decon.pdf. Accessed March 8, 2005.

[22] Hurst CG. Decontamination. In: Zajtchuk R, Bellamy RF, editors. Medical aspects of chemical and biological warfare. Washington (DC): Office of the Surgeon General, Borden Institute; 1997. p. 351–9.

[23] Wormser U, Brodsky B, Sintov A. Skin toxicokinetics of mustard gas in the guinea pig: effect of hypochlorite and safety aspects. Arch Toxicol 2002;76(9):517–22.

[24] Sidell FR, Hurst CG. Long-term health effects of nerve agent and mustard. In: Zajtchuk R, Bellamy RF, editors. Textbook of military medicine. Part I: Medical aspects of chemical and biological warfare. Falls Church (VA): Office of the Surgeon General, Dept of the Army; 1997. p. 229–46.

[25] Wils ER, Hulst AG, van Laar J. Analysis of thiodiglycol in urine of victims of an alleged attack with mustard gas, Part II. J Anal Toxicol 1988;12(1):15–9.

[26] Anderson DR, Byers SL, Vesely KR. Treatment of sulfur mustard (HD)-induced lung injury. J Appl Toxicol 2000;20(Suppl 1):S129–32.

[27] Wormser U. Protective effect of povidone iodine ointment against skin lesions induced by chemical and thermal stimuli. J Appl Toxicol 2000;20(Suppl 1):S183–5.

[28] Smith KJ, Hurst CG, Moeller RB, et al. Sulfur mustard: its continuing threat as a chemical warfare agent, the cutaneous lesions induced, progress in understanding its mechanism of action, its long-term health effects, and new developments for protection and therapy. J Am Acad Dermatol 1995;32:765–76.

[29] Hickling KG, Henderson SJ, Jackson R. Low mortality associated with low volume pressure limited ventilation with permissive hypercapnia in severe adult respiratory distress syndrome. Intensive Care Med 1990;16:372–7.

[30] Amato MB, Barbas CS, Medeiros DM, et al. Effect of a protective-ventilation strategy on mortality in the acute respiratory distress syndrome. N Engl J Med 1998;338:347–54.

[31] The Acute Respiratory Distress Network. Ventilation with lower tidal volumes as compared with traditional tidal volumes for acute lung injury and the acute respiratory distress syndrome. N Engl J Med 2000;342:1301–8.

[32] Emad A, Rezaian GR. The diversity of the effects of sulfur mustard gas inhalation on respiratory system 10 years after a single, heavy exposure: analysis of 197 cases. Chest 1997;112:734–8.

[33] Smith KJ, Hurst CG, Moeller RB, et al. Sulfur mustard: its continuing threat as a chemical warfare agent, the cutaneous lesions induced, progress in understanding its mechanism of action, its long-term health effects, and new developments for protection and therapy. J Am Acad Dermatol 1995;32(5 Pt 1):765–76.

[34] Yamakido M, Ishioka S, Hiyama K, et al. Former poison gas workers and cancer: incidence and inhibition of tumor formation by treatment with biological response modifier N-CWS. Environ Health Perspect 1996;104(Suppl 3):485–8.

[35] Safarinejad MR, Moosavi SA, Montazeri B. Ocular injuries caused by mustard gas: diagnosis, treatment, and medical defense. Mil Med 2001;166:67–70.

ELSEVIER
SAUNDERS

CRITICAL
CARE
CLINICS

Crit Care Clin 21 (2005) 719–737

Respiratory Agents: Irritant Gases, Riot Control Agents, Incapacitants, and Caustics

Craig R. Warden, MD, MPH

*Oregon Health & Science University, UHN52, Department of Emergency Medicine,
3181 SW Sam Jackson Park Road, Portland, OR 97201, USA*

The prototypical irritant gases are ammonia, chlorine, and phosgene. Chlorine and phosgene were extensively used in World War I (WWI), causing about 1.3 million casualties [1,2]. Chlorine is heavier than air, and caused severe mucosal and airway irritability, forcing soldiers to leave their trenches and thus to sustain great losses from rifle and artillery fire. Chlorine became less effective because the odor and mucosal irritation provided excellent warning properties, the development of effective gas masks, and the availability of deadlier war gases. Chlorine is extensively used in industrial processes, and transported in huge quantities. Thus, chlorine is frequently involved in unintentional releases [3–6]. There have been infrequent uses of chlorine by disgruntled employees or terrorists [7].

Phosgene became the prominent war gas in WWI, and was used frequently in combination with chlorine [2,8–11]. It was dispersed in liquid filled shells with rapid vaporization on detonation. Because phosgene was four times the density of air, it quickly settled into the trenches. There are reports of the use of phosgene by the Japanese on the Chinese during World War II (WWII), by Egypt in Yemen during 1963–1967, and by Iraq and Iran during their 1980s conflict [9]. The most significant unintentional release was in 1928, in Hamburg, Germany. The approximately 11 metric tons formed a gas cloud for 10 km, causing at least 300 casualties, including 10 deaths [12]. The Aum Shinrikyo cult used phosgene on a journalist in Yokohama, Japan, by introducing it through her apartment's mail slot, resulting in her hospitalization [12]. Diphosgene (trichoromethylchloroformate) was also used during WWI by combining chloroform and phosgene.

E-mail address: wardenc@ohsu.edu

After release, the combination breaks down into its components. The parent compound has an additional lachrymator effect [8,9].

Riot control agents

Chloroacetophenone (CN), chlorobenzylidenemalonitrile (CS), chloropicrin (PS), bromobenzylcyanide, diphenylaminearsine (DM, adamsite), dibenzoxazepine, and oleoresin capsicum (OC, "pepper spray"), along with combinations of these, have all been used at various times as riot control agents, harassing agents, or "tear gases." Ethylbromoacetate, the riot control agent originally used by French police, was actually the first "war" gas used during WWI [13,14]. During the Vietnam War, the United States used CS extensively until it was stopped by executive order [13]. Riot control agents have been used in large-scale civil disturbances, most notably in Paris, France, in 1968, in Londonderry, Northern Ireland, in 1969, and many times in America, including prison riots and most notably in Waco, Texas, where their flammability was demonstrated. CN was the standard tear gas used by most military and civilian police forces until CS was widely distributed by the 1950s [13,14]. PS also used as a fumigant. DM, the only widely stocked "vomiting agent," is not known to be currently available.

Incapacitating agents

Many conflicts have involved various nonlethal incapacitating agents dating back to antiquity using various naturally occurring anticholinergic preparations such as belladonna. Many agents have been studied as potential incapacitants such as stimulants, psychedelics, and sedative-hypnotics, none of which worked very well [9,15–17]. The only known weaponized incapacitating agent has been 3-quinuclidinyl benzilate (BZ); this agent was available in the United States stockpile (developed in the 1960s), and is known only to have been used on military "volunteers" [16–18]. Iraq apparently stockpiled an almost identical agent dubbed "Agent 15" that was found during the first Gulf War [9]. There have been allegations of the use of incapacitating agents in the twentieth century in French Indochina, Afghanistan, Mozambique, and Yugoslavia [18,19].

In October 2002, the Russian military apparently used an incapacitating agent in an attempt to free 800 hostages from a Moscow theater that was taken by Chechen terrorists. The best evidence so far points to the use of a combination of aerosolized carfentanil, a very lipophilic derivative of fentanyl, and a general anesthetic such as halothane [20–24]. Unfortunately, the special forces troops and the medical community were not prepared to handle the resulting mass casualties involved, and 127 (16%) hostages died in addition to all the terrorists. The Russian government never fully acknowledged what agents were used [24]. There are recent reports of the US military trying to weaponize drugs such as diazepam [22,25].

Caustic agents

Caustic agents include strong acids, bases, and oxidizers. There are too many available caustic agents to discuss in detail. Chemical exposures to caustics are very common, at least 100,000 are reported yearly to United States poison centers, resulting in only about 20 deaths per year [5]. Incendiary substances such as magnesium, thermite, and white phosphorus are mostly used for military purposes [26,27].

Mechanism of toxicity

Irritant gases

Proposed use as a weapon
The irritant gases are ubiquitous in many industrial processes, and are transported in huge quantities by rail and truck, thus making them easy targets for terrorism [3,4,6]. Chlorine is widely available in many locations besides factories (pools and water treatment plants), and could easily be diverted for terrorist uses.

Method of exposure
The most likely method of exposure for the irritant gases would be industrial or transportation incidents or sabotage. Almost all of the exposures would be inhalational because of the low boiling points and volatility of these compounds. Victims in the immediate vicinity of the escaping gas stream could sustain cutaneous chemical burns.

Biochemical, cellular, and systemic effects
At room temperature phosgene is a colorless, nonflammable, heavier-than-air gas with an odor of newly mown hay that is not appreciated by all people. Under 47°F (8°C), phosgene is a colorless, fuming liquid. It is shipped as a liquefied, compressed gas that can cause frostbite on contact. Phosgene's inadequate warning properties and delayed symptoms make it a potentially useful terrorist weapon [11,28]. Phosgene is only slightly soluble in water, hence its deeper penetration in the pulmonary system. On contact with water it hydrolyzes into carbon dioxide and hydrochloric acid, resulting in direct caustic damage. In addition, phosgene also undergoes acylation reactions with amino-, hydroxyl-, and sulfhydryl- groups of cellular macromolecules, resulting in cell damage and apoptosis [6,8,10,11,29–33]. The end result is damage to the alveolar-capillary membranes causing capillary leak, noncardiogenic pulmonary edema, and possibly hypovolemic shock. Phosgene is not absorbed by intact skin, and any systematic effects are secondary to anoxia [28].

Chlorine is a greenish yellow gas, an oxidizing agent, and very reactive with water. Chlorine upon contact with water liberates hypochlorous acid, hydrochloric acid, and oxygen-free radicals. It has intermediate solubility, and causes irritant effects throughout the respiratory tree but mostly in the eyes, nasal mucosa and the upper airway. Cell damage is caused by its strong oxidizing capability and release of hydrochloric acid; in addition, hypochlorous acid can penetrate cells and react with cytoplasmic proteins [4,6,10,11,32,34–36]. Chlorine has a pungent odor, and coupled with early mucosal irritation, provides the gas with excellent warning properties. These features may mitigate its effects where potential victims have routes of escape. However, prolonged exposure may lead to olfactory fatigue and compromise the evacuation effort. Even low-concentration exposures can increase airway resistance in both normal and airway hyperresponsive subjects [37].

At room temperature, anhydrous ammonia is a colorless, highly irritating gas with a very pungent odor that is lighter than air. It is easily compressed for transportation and storage to form a clear, colorless liquid that, upon release, will initially be heavier than air. Ammonia readily dissolves in water to form ammonium hydroxide, a very caustic alkaline solution, accounting for its mechanism of injury [38–40]. Ammonia also has excellent warning properties, but if escape is not immediate, it too can cause olfactory fatigue and more prolonged exposure [41].

Riot control agents

Proposed use as a weapon

Riot control agents are generally disseminated by explosive dispersion of the powder or solution, spraying fine droplets or particles or by releasing as a smoke from a pyrotechnic mixture, and have been used frequently in small-scale exposures such in building air vents [7].

Method of exposure

Most exposures are inhalational, ocular, or dermal.

Biochemical, cellular, and systemic effects

CS and CN are white, crystalline solids with a low vapor pressure and low water solubility [13]. CN requires a higher concentration to be effective, is more toxic, and a more potent dermal sensitizer than CS [13,42]. Typical exposures lead to eye, nose, and throat irritation, leading to immediate behavior to escape [14,43–47]. High-dose exposures in an enclosed space may lead to airway edema, noncardiogenic pulmonary edema, and possibly respiratory arrest [48–51]. CS is a primary irritant to the skin, and individuals can develop an allergic contact dermatitis to subsequent exposures [43,44]. Life-threatening effects and death from noncardiogenic pulmonary edema have been documented with indiscriminate use of CN in confined spaces but not with CS [13,49,51]. DM is a yellow-green, odorless, crystalline compound that causes delayed lacrimator symptoms including uncontrollable sneezing and coughing, and also has prolonged systemic effects with headache, malaise, nausea, abdominal cramps, vomiting, and diarrhea [14]. These factors would add to the incapacitation and panic in the civilian population. OC is a mixture of many chemicals extracted from chili peppers that acts on many pathways including Substance P, causing intense burning pain, tearing, neurogenic inflammation, and edema in the eyes and burning pain and erythema of the skin [14,52,53].

Incapacitating agents

Proposed use as a weapon
The various incapacitating agents would be most likely be used by legal authorities in hostage situations. They may find use by terrorists to induce panic and overwhelm the medical system [15–17]. It is possible to disperse BZ-like agents in the food supply due to its persistence. Fentanyl derivatives and benzodiazepines would need to be aerosolized for large-scale use [20,23–25].

Method of exposure
BZ-like agents could be dispersed as an aerosolized solid for primary inhalation absorption or dissolved in a solvent for ingestion or dermal absorption.

Biochemical, cellular, and systemic effects
BZ is an odorless, nonirritating glycolate anticholinergic agent related to atropine, scopolamine, and hyoscyamine. It acts as a competitive acetylcholine inhibitor at postsynaptic and postjunctional muscarinic receptors in smooth muscle, exocrine glands, autonomic ganglia, and brain. It has a very large physiologic safety ratio, but victims might endanger themselves secondary to paranoid hallucinations. The fentanyl derivatives act primarily on the various central nervous system (CNS) opioid receptors causing lethargy, respiratory depression, and miosis. Benzodiazepines work on CNS gamma-aminobutyric acid receptors causing sedation, lethargy, and eventually coma and respiratory depression.

Caustic agents

Proposed use as a weapon
Just like the irritant gases, huge quantities of common caustics such as hydrochloric acid, sulfuric acid, hydrofluoric acid, chromic acid, nitric acid, sodium hydroxide, phenol, concentrated hypochlorite solutions, and white and red phosphorus are stored and transported throughout America. Well-executed sabotage at a fixed facility or transport corridor could create mass casualties and panic. On the other hand, unintentional incidents involving these substances occur so frequently that hazardous material (HAZMAT) responses should mitigate circumstances. Incendiary devices could be diverted from military sources.

Method of exposure
Most exposures will be inhalational in a large release. Patients closer to the release may have dermal exposure causing burns. Most caustics have excellent warning properties, allowing escape to minimize exposure. Incendiary devices

would most likely produce dermal burns without significant inhalational injury unless used in a confined space.

Biochemical, cellular, and systemic effects

Acids and bases combine with their cellular counterparts producing an exothermic reaction. All of the caustics cause airway injury through direct cell injury leading to necrosis, edema, and increased secretions. Alkali substances produce a liquefaction necrosis that typically allows deeper penetration, while acids produce a coagulation necrosis that helps to limit the depth of the burn. A significant hydrofluoric acid exposure can lead to fluoride binding of calcium and magnesium leading to dysrhythmias [54]. Incendiaries such as magnesium, white phosphorus (which spontaneously ignites on exposure to air), and thermite (a mixture of granular aluminum and iron oxide) cause both a thermal and oxidative injury, leading to cell necrosis [26]. Enough white phosphorus could be absorbed dermally to produce hypocalcemia, with tetany and characteristic EKG changes (prolonged QT interval, ST segment depression, and T-wave changes) and dysrhythmias [26,27,55].

Clinical presentation

Irritant gases

Symptoms and sequence of symptoms

Phosgene has delayed effects from 20 minutes up to 48 hours, depending on the intensity of exposure and subsequent physical activity of the victim. The shorter the latency period, the worse the prognosis [6,8,11,28,29,32]. Initial upper airway irritant symptoms (eye irritation, rhinorrhea, cough) are usually mild, but depend on the intensity of exposure with significant symptoms indicating a worse exposure. The patient then will develop lower respiratory symptoms with shortness of breath, substernal burning, and chest tightness [31,33]. On physical examination, the patient may exhibit fine basilar crackles and wheezing and worsening hypoxemia. As pulmonary edema becomes more evident, the patient will exhibit coarser crackles and production of watery frothy white or yellow pulmonary secretions. The development of overt pulmonary edema within 4 hours of exposure portends a poor prognosis, and aggressive critical care is required to avert death [10,11,56,57]. Secondary bacterial pulmonary infections can become evident in 4 to 5 days. Radiographs of the chest early in the course can demonstrate hyperinflation progressing to a picture of noncardiogenic pulmonary edema.

Typical accidental exposures to chlorine gas result in eye and nasopharyngeal irritation with tearing, rhinorrhea, sneezing, and hypersalivation, along with psychologic symptoms associated with fear or panic [4,34]. Higher levels of exposure causing lower airway injury will result in cough, shortness of breath, retrosternal chest pain, and systematic complaints of headache, nausea, vomiting, and lightheadedness [6,10,11,32,35]. Corneal burns and dermal irritation may occur with splash or high concentration exposures. Patients will exhibit tachypnea, tachycardia, wheezing, chest wall retractions, signs of laryngeal edema and laryngospasm, lacrimation, and blepharospasm [3,35,36].

Ammonia is the prototypical highly water-soluble irritant and caustic agent causing primarily upper airway symptoms. Even low concentrations cause rapid eye and nose irritation with higher concentrations causing corneal injuries [38,40]. Concentrated ammonia solutions (25%) can cause severe corrosive injury to intact skin, eyes, and gastrointestinal tract. Upper airway edema and lower airway injury can occur with exposure to high concentrations or inability to escape. Upper airway obstruction is the immediate cause of death; in addition, patients can develop tracheobronchial burns and noncardiogenic pulmonary edema.

Differential diagnosis
See Table 1.

Estimate of number of potential critical care patients
Ammonia and chlorine open air exposures with adequate escape routes should result in relatively few critical patients. Phosgene due to its poor warning properties could cause large numbers of critically ill patients [10].

Riot control agents

Symptoms and sequence of symptoms
Exposure to riot control agents causes immediate irritant effects on the eyes and nasal mucosa, with intense lacrimation, blepharospasm, rhinorrhea, burning sensations of nose and eyes, and conjunctival injection [13,43,44,46,47]. Exposed skin can develop redness and pain [42,58]. More intense exposures will cause oropharyngeal irritation and injection, sore throat, coughing, dysphonia, salivation, and dysphagia. Patients may also manifest chest tightness, shortness of breath, and wheezing [50]. Serious eye injuries can occur from the explosive force or clumping and embedding in the cornea of solid residual particles [13,45]. The mucosal effects of riot control agents are usually short lived (15–30 minutes) after the patient has been removed from the source and decontaminated. Skin symptoms such as erythema and burning sensation can last up to 45 to 60 minutes after cessation of exposure [59,60]. More prolonged symptoms should prompt the search for possible other exposures or underlying comorbidities such as asthma. OC acts in a similar fashion, but has more airway sensitizing potential [14,52,53].

Differential diagnosis
See Table 1.

Table 1
Differential diagnosis of respiratory agents

	Irritant gases	Riot control agents	Incapacitants	Caustics
Substance characteristics	Visible clouds, heavier than air Good warning properties (except phosgene)	Dispersed as explosive powder or aerosol cloud (white)	Aerosol or in solvent for food Odorless, nonirritating	Liquid or vapor clouds Incendiary: pyrotechnic, residual particulate matter Good warning properties (except HF)
Time course	Rapid onset (except phosgene) Short duration unless develop NPE Phosgene: shorter the onset, the worse the prognosis	Immediate Short duration unless in confined space	BZ delayed onset of 30 min to 4 hr BZ duration 48–72 h Narcotic/sedative short onset and duration	Rapid onset Significant exposure: prolonged symptoms HF can have delayed symptoms
Symptoms	Mucosal and upper airway irritation prominent Severe: dyspnea	Severe tearing, eye pain, nasal burning Cough Skin irritation	BZ: agitation, hallucinations, dry mouth, blurry vision Narcotic/sedative: confusion, lethargy, initial euphoria	Immediate mucosal and upper airway irritation (except HF) Dermal burns

Signs	Rhinorrhea, tearing Bronchospasm NPE: crackles, cyanosis, ↑WOB	Ocular, nasal, and throat irritation prominent Cough NPE: extremely rare	BZ: anticholinergic syndrome Narcotic/sedative: lethargy, coma, respiratory depression, miosis	Dermal burns prominent Alkali: liquefaction necrosis Acids: coagulation necrosis Upper airway injury prominent
Response to antidotes	None	None	BZ: physostigmine clears sensorium Fentanyl-like substances: naloxone awakens Benzodiazepines: flumazenil awakens	Calcium for HF: reduces symptoms, reverses EKG changes
Labs	None diagnostic ABG to document respiratory status	None helpful or diagnostic	None helpful Drug screens might be positive	Monitor Ca/Mg in HF Monitor Ca in white phosphorus burns
Imaging	CXR: "batwing" infiltrates, normal heart size in NPE	Should be negative unless rare NPE	Not helpful unless possible aspiration from coma	NPE on CXR if significant exposure

Abbreviations: BZ, 3-quinuclidinyl benzilate; CXR, chest radiograph; HF, hydrofluoric acid; NPE, noncardiogenic pulmonary edema; WOB, work of breathing.

Estimate of number of potential critical care patients

Riot control exposures should not produce any critical care patients unless used in a confined space with prolonged exposure [51].

Incapacitating agents

Symptoms and sequence of symptoms

Onset of symptoms after exposure to BZ usually starts in 30 minutes to 4 hours, but may not be manifest in up to 20 hours [15,17,18]. CNS effects range from stupor, confusion with short-term memory loss, and short attention span, ataxia, seizures, agitated delirium, visual hallucinations, and repetitive behavior. Peripheral effects would include mydriasis, decreased visual acuity, decreased sweating, flushed skin, decreased gastrointestinal motility, bladder distension, tachycardia, hypertension, and hyperthermia ("dry as a bone, blind as a bat, red as a beet, hot as a hare, crazy as a hatter"). Symptoms may last up to 72 to 96 hours in a dose-dependent fashion [15].

The fentanyl derivatives, especially the very lipophylic ones, in an inhaled aerosolized form would have a very rapid onset of action making it a potentially effective incapacitating agent for law enforcement with the appropriate medical rescue preparation [20–24]. In large enough doses patients would be unconscious soon after noticing the euphoric effects. Benzodiazepines theoretically would have similar effects, but have not been tested [25].

Differential diagnosis

See Table 1.

Estimate of number of potential critical care patients

A large number of casualties could be generated with the use of BZ. One would not expect a large component of exposed patients to need critical care once adequate sedation is achieved. The use of an opioid or benzodiazepine-based incapacitating agent could produce a large number of critical patients even if antidotes are available in large quantities. A large number of patients could prevent quick resuscitation and administration of antidote creating patients with anoxic brain injuries.

Caustic agents

Symptoms and sequence of symptoms

All of the caustics except for possibly hydrofluoric acid (HF) would cause immediate symptoms when inhaled, and the acids and bases that are water soluble will have prominent ocular, nasal, and upper airway symptoms similar to ammonia [54]. Patients exposed to high concentrations or trapped in confined spaces could develop noncardiogenic pulmonary edema. Significant exposures to

HF may lead to hypocalcemia and hypomagnesium, with symptoms of tetany, dysrhythmias, and cardiac arrest. Patients may also have prominent dermal burns in these circumstances or if exposed directly to liquid. Incendiary exposure would most likely cause dermal burns, but could cause inhalation injury if used in a confined space [26,27,55].

Differential diagnosis
See Table 1.

Estimate of number of potential critical care patients
If a concentrated exposure is achieved in a large crowd there could be many critical patients. In typical HAZMAT situations seen with these substances there are relatively few critical patients unless some are trapped.

Decontamination in the emergency department and intensive care unit

Specific issues/cautions
There is still evidence that hospitals are woefully unprepared for contaminated patients [61,62]. Because exposure to most of these agents will be inhalational, there is little risk of secondary contamination or off-gassing for hospital personnel [12,63–65]. Prudent field decontamination should include undressing and brief water decontamination before transport [66–69]. If there is any liquid exposure, more prolonged irrigation should be used. The same decontamination procedure should be done in the emergency department if not accomplished before arrival [68]. Caustic exposures may involve more contamination risk, depending on circumstances, and will require more prolonged irrigation. For patients who present with known exposure to one of these agents but undecontaminated to the hospital, Level C protection (full-face mask with powered canister filtration with chemical-resistant gown, gloves, and boots) would be prudent [70]. If substance is unknown or patient is heavily contaminated, Level B protection (hose-supplied air or SCBA) may be necessary [64,71,72].

HF dermal exposures should be decontaminated with calcium or magnesium containing fluids or gels [54]. CS and CN should be decontaminated with water, alkaline soap and water, or a mildly alkaline solution of sodium bicarbonate, sodium carbonate, or benzalkonium chloride, and specifically not hypochlorite solutions [13,58]. Residual particulate matter of incendiary substances should be removed completely before water irrigation to prevent further thermal injury (this is less of an issue with thermite) [26,55]. These agents have significant secondary contamination potential.

Isolation if appropriate
Patients exposed to any of these agents will not need to be isolated once adequately decontaminated.

Diagnostic studies

Screening

All patients should receive chest radiography to look for signs of non-cardiogenic pulmonary edema and other causes of their respiratory distress (pneumothorax, hemothorax, pneumonia). Other tests will depend on the patient's presentation and severity of illness. Continuous pulse oximetry is helpful in titrating oxygen therapy and deciding on the use of positive airway pressure and intubation. Blood gases can confirm acid-base status and adequacy of ventilation. Monitoring expiratory flow rates may help guide bronchodilator therapy and need for more aggressive airway support. Routine blood work such as complete blood counts and chemistry panels are usually not helpful in the early stages of the exposure but may become abnormal as the patient develops pulmonary edema and hypovolemia. All patients should be screened for traumatic injuries secondary to blasts or occurring during escape (falls, trampling).

Definitive

Laryngoscopy and bronchoscopy may be helpful in assessing airway compromise in the irritant gas or caustic exposure and clearing airway debris and secretions. Exposure to the irritant gases should be delineated by characteristics of gas itself, length of onset of symptoms, and relative involvement of upper versus lower airways. Exposure to anticholinergic, benzodiazepine, or narcotic-based incapacitating agents should be readily diagnosed by their toxidromes and response to antidotes (below). There is variability in the capability of routine urine drug screens to pick up synthetic opioids and some benzodiazepines. Patients with a significant exposure to hydrofluoric acid or white phosphorus need serial monitoring of serum electrolytes including calcium and magnesium and continuous cardiac monitoring for dysrhythmias.

Antidotes

There are no specific antidotes for the irritant gases, riot control agents, or most of the caustic agents. There has been anecdotal use of nebulized sodium bicarbonate for chlorine exposures, despite a theoretic concern for producing a mucosal exothermic reaction [73]. Similarly, HF respiratory, and ocular exposures have been anecdotally treated with nebulized or irrigant containing calcium gluconate, respectively, with no clear improved outcome [54,74]. If there is significant dermal exposure and absorption, intravenous or intra-arterial calcium gluconate may be needed.

The anticholinergic incapacitating agents can be treated with titratable doses of physostigmine to help clarify the diagnosis and treat symptoms. Unfortunately, physostigmine's duration of action is usually much shorter than the anticholinergic agents, and sedation with benzodiazepines should be used to control persistent patient agitation [59]. Physostigmine used indiscriminately can cause a cholinergic syndrome similar to the nerve agents, and has lead to patient deaths [75]. Any of the narcotic or benzodiazepine-based incapacitating agents can be treated easily with naloxone or flumazenil, respectively, if given before onset of anoxic brain injury.

Supportive care

Irritant gases

The primary focus in treating exposures to any of the irritant gases is airway and ventilation support. Because exertion is known to increase the toxicity, casualties need enforced bed rest [11]. High concentration exposures including phosgene can result in upper airway edema and laryngospasm, resulting in early mortality. Any significant upper airway symptoms such as stridor mandates early intubation. Provide supplementary oxygen and airway suctioning for excess secretions. Bronchospasm should be treated with inhaled beta agonists such as albuterol and anticholinergic agents such as ipratropium. Early signs of pulmonary edema may be managed with continuous positive away pressure or bilevel positive airway pressure. Diuretics are not indicated, and in fact, patients may be hypovolemic from capillary leak. Patients are susceptible to positive airway pressure-induced hypotension requiring isotonic fluid administration. Inotropes are not usually needed if adequate fluid resuscitation is maintained. Steroids are not indicated for irritant gas exposures unless significant reactive airway disease is evident [11]. Intubation with positive end-expiratory pressure will be frequently required, and should be the primary means of airway support in a patient with any poor prognostic indicators as discussed above [6,10,11,29, 32,38,39,76–78]. Blind nasotracheal intubation or use of an esophageal obturator is discouraged because of the risk of disrupting severely injured mucosa [28,41,79]. There is no evidence to support the use of prophylactic antibiotics. Bacterial superinfection can become evident 4 to 5 days after exposure, and should be treated with appropriate antibiotics guided by clinical specimens.

Riot control agents

After removal from exposure including disrobing and decontamination with ocular and skin irrigation, no further treatment is usually required. Symptomatic treatment may include analgesics and antipruritics. Except for OC, there is no evidence that the common riot control agents such as CS and CN affect pulmonary functions with typical exposures [13,14]. For the unusual exposures of high doses in confined spaces, the supportive care outlined for the irritant gases is appropriate. There is no evidence of permanent sequelae. OC can cause bronchoconstriction, increased secretions, and airway edema in normal patients.

In conditions of high a concentration of the agent, high temperature, and high humidity, there has been evidence of a more severe dermatitis, leading to vesication [13,14]. These skin injuries should be treated as usual burn injuries. For persistently erythematous intact skin, topical steroids are useful [13].

Incapacitating agents

Supportive care is usually necessary even with the availability of antidotes. For the anticholinergic agents, physostigmine can be used both to diagnose and treat the anticholinergic delirium [75]. Patients generally need to be sedated generously with benzodiazepines to treat agitated delirium with its attendant hyperthermia, rhabdomyolysis, and potential harm from physical restraint [15–17,59]. Intravenous fluids should be given to treat dehydration and promote diuresis of myoglobin. Standard treatment for rhabdomyolysis should be instituted. Seizures need to be treated aggressively to prevent hyperthermia and CNS injury.

If a narcotic or benzodiazepine-based agent is suspected, aggressive airway and ventilatory support will be needed until appropriate antidotes can be administered, both of which may be difficult to achieve in a mass casualty situation [23,24].

Caustic agents

Once decontaminated, supportive care for respiratory exposures should proceed as for irritant gases above. Burn care is the same as for thermal burns [26,55]. Hydrofluoric acid exposures may require nebulized, topical, intravenous, or intra-arterial calcium gluconate to counter its calcium binding toxicity [54,74]. White phosphorus burns may allow absorption causing hypocalcemia that may require calcium replacement [27].

Clinical course and prognostic factors

Irritant gases

If the patient survives the initial 48 hours after exposure to phosgene, survival is likely [11,28,41,76,77,79,80]. Sensitivity to irritants can persist, resulting in the reactive airway dysfunction syndrome with bronchospasm and chronic airway inflammation. Tissue destruction and scarring can lead to bronchiectasis, lobar emphysema, atelectasis, and recurrent pulmonary infections [11,28,41, 76,77,79,80]. In a large occupational exposure during WWII in a uranium-processing plant, 106 male workers were exposed to high levels of phosgene, resulting in 24% developing acute pneumonitis on radiologic examination with only one dying [56,57]. Patients who remain asymptomatic after 6 hours can be discharged safely home with explicit instructions to return for any subsequent symptoms. This is especially important in a mass casualty situation to preserve bedspace. The onset of symptoms after 6 hours is usually gradual with adequate time to return for treatment [11,28].

Morbidity and mortality from chlorine exposures result for noncardiogenic pulmonary edema. This may occur within 2 to 4 hours of exposure at moderate concentrations but within 30 to 60 minutes of severe exposures [3,36]. Pulmonary function usually returns to baseline within 7 to 14 days, but patients may have long-term sequelae including reactive airway dysfunction syndrome [30,81,82]. Asymptomatic patients (except for some ocular or nasal irritation) can be watched for 6 hours, and if no signs of pulmonary edema are evident, can be released home to return for any pulmonary symptoms [11,35]. Otherwise, symptomatic patients should be watched for complete resolution of symptoms.

Survivors of severe ammonia exposure can have residual chronic lung disease with scarring [38]. Ulceration and perforation of the cornea can occur weeks after the exposure, along with cataracts and glaucoma. Ingestions can cause perforations and residual scarring causing dysmotility and obstruction.

Riot control agents

Only patients with severe underlying pulmonary disease or with a high concentration exposure in an enclosed space need to be observed for the development of lower airway involvement. There is no evidence of long-term effects from exposure to CS or CN, but there may be long-term sensitization to OC [14,44,46,48,52]. Other patients only need symptomatic care with analgesics or antipruritics.

Incapacitating agents

Patients exposed to an anticholinergic incapacitating agents can be symptomatic for several days. Once adequately sedated and monitored and treated for the sequelae of hyperthermia and rhabdomyolysis, patients should have a relatively benign course. Due to the severe respiratory suppression possible with the narcotic, benzodiazepine, or general anesthetic-based agents, patients may have significant anoxic brain injury after initial resuscitation and require prolonged ventilatory support [20,21,23,24].

Caustic agents

Most injury from the caustics will peak soon after exposure. Noncardiogenic pulmonary edema should be evident within hours of exposure. Dermal burns should also be evident early in the course. The exception may be exposure to hydrofluoric acid, which, depending on the concentration, may manifest in a delayed fashion [54]. Incendiary agents can produce burns that will need long-term care and pulmonary injury similar to the irritant agents if used in a confined space [27].

References

[1] Bismuth C, Borron SW, Baud FJ, et al. Chemical weapons: documented use and compounds on the horizon. Toxicol Lett 2004;149(1–3):11–8.

[2] Eckert WG. Mass deaths by gas or chemical poisoning. A historical perspective. Am J Forensic Med Pathol 1991;12(2):119–25.

[3] Blanc PD, Galbo M, Hiatt P, et al. Morbidity following acute irritant inhalation in a population-based study. JAMA 1991;266(5):664–9.

[4] Winder C. The toxicology of chlorine. Environ Res 2001;85(2):105–14.

[5] Watson WA, Litovitz TL, Klein-Schwartz W, et al. 2003 annual report of the American Association of Poison Control Centers Toxic Exposure Surveillance System. Am J Emerg Med 2004;22(5):335–404.

[6] Rorison DG, McPherson SJ. Acute toxic inhalations. Emerg Med Clin North Am 1992;10(2): 409–35.

[7] Turnbull W, Abhayaratne P. 2002 WMD terrorism chronology: incidents involving sub-national actors and chemical, biological, radiological, and nuclear materials. Monterey, CA: Center for Nonproliferation Studies, Monterey Institute of International Studies; 2003.

[8] Compton J. Diphosgene. In: Compton J, editor. Military chemical and biological agents: chemical and toxicological properties. Caldwell (NJ): Telford Press; 1987. p. 124–34.

[9] Smart J. History of chemical and biological warfare. In: Sidell FR, Takafuji ET, Franz DR, editors. Medical aspects of chemical and biological warfare. 3rd edition. Washington (DC): Government Printing Office; 1997. p. 9–86.

[10] Urbanetti J. Toxic Inhalational Injury. In: Sidell FR, Takafuji ET, Franz DR, editors. Medical aspects of chemical and biological warfare. 3rd edition. Washington (DC): Government Printing Office; 1997. p. 247–70.

[11] Pulmonary agents. In: US Army medical research institute of chemical defense, medical management of chemical casualties handbook. 3rd edition. Aberdeen (MA): USAMRICD; 2000. p. 18–34.

[12] Lazarus AA, Devereaux A. Potential agents of chemical warfare. Worst-case scenario protection and decontamination methods. Postgrad Med 2002;112(5):133–40.

[13] Sidell F. Riot control agents. In: Sidell FR, Takafuji ET, Franz DR, editors. Medical aspects of chemical and biological warfare. 3rd edition. Washington (DC): Government Printing Office; 1997. p. 307–24.

[14] Olajos EJ, Salem H. Riot control agents: pharmacology, toxicology, biochemistry and chemistry. J Appl Toxicol 2001;21(5):355–91.

[15] Ketchum JS, Sidell FR. Incapacitating agents. In: Sidell FR, Takafuji ET, Franz DR, editors. Medical aspects of chemical and biological warfare. 3rd edition. Washington (DC): Government Printing Office; 1997. p. 287–305.

[16] Chemical casualties. Sensory incapacitants. J R Army Med Corps 2002;148(4):392–4.

[17] Chemical casualties. Centrally acting incapacitants. J R Army Med Corps 2002;148(4): 388–91.

[18] Incapacitating agents. In: US Army medical research institute of chemical defense, medical management of chemical casualties handbook. 3rd edition. Aberdeen (MA): USAMRICD; 2000. p. 124–53.

[19] Hay A. Surviving the impossible: the long march from Srebrenica. An investigation of the possible use of chemical warfare agents. Med Confl Surviv 1998;14(2):120–55.

[20] Rieder J, Keller C, Hoffmann G, et al. Moscow theatre siege and anaesthetic drugs. Lancet 2003;361(9363):1131.

[21] Coupland RM. Incapacitating chemical weapons: a year after the Moscow theatre siege. Lancet 2003;362(9393):1346.

[22] Schiermeier Q. Hostage deaths put gas weapons in spotlight. Nature 2002;420(6911):7.

[23] Enserink M, Stone R. Toxicology. Questions swirl over knockout gas used in hostage crisis. Science 2002;298(5596):1150–1.

[24] Wax PM, Becker CE, Curry SC. Unexpected "gas" casualties in Moscow: a medical toxicology perspective. Ann Emerg Med 2003;41(5):700–5.

[25] Stone A. Chemical weapons. US research on sedatives in combat sets off alarms. Science 2002; 297(5582):764.

[26] Chemical casualties. Smokes, fuels, and incendiary materials. J R Army Med Corps 2002; 148(4):395–7.

[27] Konjoyan TR. White phosphorus burns: case report and literature review. Mil Med 1983; 148(11):881–4.

[28] Medical management guideline for phosgene. Managing hazardous material incidents, volume III: agency for toxic substances and disease registry. Atlanta (GA): US Department of Health and Human Services; 2001.

[29] Borak J, Diller WF. Phosgene exposure: mechanisms of injury and treatment strategies. J Occup Environ Med 2001;43(2):110–9.

[30] Karalliedde L, Wheeler H, Maclehose R, et al. Possible immediate and long-term health effects following exposure to chemical warfare agents. Public Health 2000;114(4):238–48.

[31] Lim SC, Yang JY, Jang AS, et al. Acute lung injury after phosgene inhalation. Korean J Intern Med 1996;11(1):87–92.

[32] Parrish JS, Bradshaw DA. Toxic inhalational injury: gas, vapor and vesicant exposure. Respir Care Clin N Am 2004;10(1):43–58.

[33] Wyatt JP, Allister CA. Occupational phosgene poisoning: a case report and review. J Accid Emerg Med 1995;12(3):212–3.

[34] Salisbury DA, Enarson DA, Chan-Yeung M, et al. First-aid reports of acute chlorine gassing among pulpmill workers as predictors of lung health consequences. Am J Ind Med 1991; 20(1):71–81.

[35] Das R, Blanc PD. Chlorine gas exposure and the lung: a review. Toxicol Ind Health 1993; 9(3):439–55.

[36] Blanc PD, Galbo M, Hiatt P, et al. Symptoms, lung function, and airway responsiveness following irritant inhalation. Chest 1993;103(6):1699–705.

[37] D'Alessandro A, Kuschner W, Wong H, et al. Exaggerated responses to chlorine inhalation among persons with nonspecific airway hyperreactivity. Chest 1996;109(2):331–7.

[38] Leung CM, Foo CL. Mass ammonia inhalational burns—experience in the management of 12 patients. Ann Acad Med Singapore 1992;21(5):624–9.

[39] Kerstein MD, Schaffzin DM, Hughes WB, et al. Acute management of exposure to liquid ammonia. Mil Med 2001;166(10):913–4.

[40] Sundblad BM, Larsson BM, Acevedo F, et al. Acute respiratory effects of exposure to ammonia on healthy persons. Scand J Work Environ Health 2004;30(4):313–21.

[41] Medical management guideline for chlorine. Managing hazardous material incidents, volume III: agency for toxic substances and disease registry. Atlanta (GA): US Department of Health and Human Services; 2001.

[42] Penneys NS, Israel RM, Indgin SM. Contact dermatitis due to 1-chloroacetophenone and chemical mace. N Engl J Med 1969;281:413–5.

[43] Anderson PJ, Lau GS, Taylor WR, et al. Acute effects of the potent lacrimator o-chlorobenzylidene malononitrile (CS) tear gas. Hum Exp Toxicol 1996;15(6):461–5.

[44] Blain PG. Tear gases and irritant incapacitants. 1-Chloroacetophenone, 2-chlorobenzylidene malononitrile and dibenz[b,f]-1,4-oxazepine. Toxicol Rev 2003;22(2):103–10.

[45] Ballantyne B, Gazzard MF, Swanston DW, et al. The ophthalmic toxicology of o-chlorobenzylidene malononitrile (CS). Arch Toxicol 1974;32(3):149–68.

[46] Karagama YG, Newton JR, Newbegin CJ. Short-term and long-term physical effects of exposure to CS spray. J R Soc Med 2003;96(4):172–4.

[47] Riot control agents. In: Division USAMRIoCDCCC, editor. Medical management of chemical casualties handbook. 3rd edition. Maclean (VA): International Book Publishing; 2000. p. 154–67.

[48] Hu H, Christiani D. Reactive airways dysfunction after exposure to teargas. Lancet 1992; 339(8808):1535.

[49] Chapman AJ, White C. Death resulting from lacrimatory agents. J Forensic Sci 1978;23(3): 527–30.

[50] Thomas RJ, Smith PA, Rascona DA, et al. Acute pulmonary effects from o-chlorobenzylidenemalonitrile "tear gas": a unique exposure outcome unmasked by strenuous exercise after a military training event. Mil Med 2002;167(2):136–9.

[51] Thorburn KM. Injuries after use of the lacrimatory agent chloroacetophenone in a confined space. Arch Environ Health 1982;37(3):182–6.

[52] Chan TC, Vilke GM, Clausen J, et al. The effect of oleoresin capsicum "pepper" spray inhalation on respiratory function. J Forensic Sci 2002;47(2):299–304.

[53] Watson WA, Stremel KR, Westdorp EJ. Oleoresin capsicum (Cap-Stun) toxicity from aerosol exposure. Ann Pharmacother 1996;30(7–8):733–5.

[54] Bertolini JC. Hydrofluoric acid: a review of toxicity. J Emerg Med 1992;10(2):163–8.

[55] Mendelson JA. Some principles of protection against burns from flame and incendiary munitions. J Trauma 1971;11(4):286–94.

[56] Polednak AP. Mortality among men occupationally exposed to phosgene in 1943–1945. Environ Res 1980;22(2):357–67.

[57] Polednak AP, Hollis DR. Mortality and causes of death among workers exposed to phosgene in 1943–45. Toxicol Ind Health 1985;1(2):137–51.

[58] Weigand D. Cutaneous reaction to the riot control agent CS. Mil Med 1969;134:437–40.

[59] Burns MJ, Linden CH, Graudins A, et al. A comparison of physostigmine and benzodiazepines for the treatment of anticholinergic poisoning. Ann Emerg Med 2000;35(4):374–81.

[60] Zekri AM, King WW, Yeung R, et al. Acute mass burns caused by o-chlorobenzylidene malononitrile (CS) tear gas. Burns 1995;21(8):586–9.

[61] Treat KN, Williams JM, Furbee PM, et al. Hospital preparedness for weapons of mass destruction incidents: an initial assessment. Ann Emerg Med 2001;38(5):562–5.

[62] Wetter DC, Daniell WE, Treser CD. Hospital preparedness for victims of chemical or biological terrorism. Am J Public Health 2001;91(5):710–6.

[63] Horton DK, Berkowitz Z, Kaye WE. Secondary contamination of ED personnel from hazardous materials events, 1995–2001. Am J Emerg Med 2003;21(3):199–204.

[64] Macintyre AG, Christopher GW, Eitzen Jr E, et al. Weapons of mass destruction events with contaminated casualties: effective planning for health care facilities. JAMA 2000;283(2): 242–9.

[65] Munro NB, Watson AP, Ambrose KR, et al. Treating exposure to chemical warfare agents: implications for health care providers and community emergency planning. Environ Health Perspect 1990;89:205–15.

[66] Bozeman WP, Dilbero D, Schauben JL. Biologic and chemical weapons of mass destruction. Emerg Med Clin North Am 2002;20(4):975–93.

[67] Biological and chemical terrorism: strategic plan for preparedness and response. Recommendations of the CDC Strategic Planning Workgroup. MMWR Recomm Rep 2000;49(RR-4): 1–14.

[68] Brennan RJ, Waeckerle JF, Sharp TW, et al. Chemical warfare agents: emergency medical and emergency public health issues. Ann Emerg Med 1999;34(2):191–204.

[69] Evison D, Hinsley D, Rice P. Chemical weapons. BMJ 2002;324(7333):332–5.

[70] Geiling JA. Role of the pulmonary provider in a terrorist attack: resources and command and control issues. Respir Care Clin N Am 2004;10(1):23–41.

[71] Arad M, Epstein Y, Krasner E, et al. Principles of respiratory protection. Isr J Med Sci 1991; 27(11–12):636–42.

[72] Heller O, Aldar Y, Vosk M, Shemer J. An argument for equipping civilian hospitals with a multiple respirator system for a chemical warfare mass casualty situation. Isr J Med Sci 1991; 27(11–12):652–5.

[73] Vinsel PJ. Treatment of acute chlorine gas inhalation with nebulized sodium bicarbonate. J Emerg Med 1990;8(3):327–9.

[74] Lee DC, Wiley 2nd JF, Synder 2nd JW. Treatment of inhalational exposure to hydrofluoric acid with nebulized calcium gluconate. J Occup Med 1993;35(5):470.

[75] Schneir AB, Offerman SR, Ly BT, et al. Complications of diagnostic physostigmine administration to emergency department patients. Ann Emerg Med 2003;42(1):14–9.

[76] Diller WF. Therapeutic strategy in phosgene poisoning. Toxicol Ind Health 1985;1(2):93–9.

[77] Diller WF, Zante R. A literature review: therapy for phosgene poisoning. Toxicol Ind Health 1985;1(2):117–28.

[78] Regan RA. Review of clinical experience in handling phosgene exposure cases. Toxicol Ind Health 1985;1(2):69–72.

[79] Medical management guideline for ammonia. Managing hazardous material incidents, volume III: agency for toxic substances and disease registry. Atlanta (GA): Department of Health and Human Services; 2001.

[80] Diller WF. Late sequelae after phosgene poisoning: a literature review. Toxicol Ind Health 1985;1(2):129–36.

[81] Schonhofer B, Voshaar T, Kohler D. Long-term lung sequelae following accidental chlorine gas exposure. Respiration (Herrlisheim) 1996;63(3):155–9.

[82] Kennedy SM, Enarson DA, Janssen RG, et al. Lung health consequences of reported accidental chlorine gas exposures among pulpmill workers. Am Rev Respir Dis 1991;143(1):74–9.

ELSEVIER
SAUNDERS

Crit Care Clin 21 (2005) 739–746

CRITICAL
CARE
CLINICS

Smallpox

Sarah D. Nafziger, MD

Department of Emergency Medicine, University of Alabama at Birmingham,
619 19ʰ Street South Jefferson Tower North 266, Birmingham, AL 35249-7013, USA

In our modern world, it is difficult to imagine that smallpox has been one of the most feared diseases throughout history; a disease that has decimated entire populations at a time. There is no natural animal reservoir or vector for variola, the virus responsible for smallpox infection. Because transmission of this disease is through person-to-person contact, outbreaks of smallpox have followed the course of human migration and travel for thousands of years. Fortunately, in 1796, Edward Jenner observed that milkmaids who had contracted cowpox, now known to be an orthopox virus similar to variola, had a lower incidence of smallpox infection. Theorizing that infectious material from an individual with a milder disease could induce a protective response against a more severe disease, Jenner is credited with developing the first smallpox vaccine. Using bovine serum containing the cowpox virus, Jenner successfully tested his vaccine, and from this discovery vaccination efforts blossomed worldwide. His bovine experiment will live on in infamy, as the word vaccination was actually coined from *vacca*, the Latin word for cow.

After the World Health Organization (WHO) began a monumental vaccination campaign in 1956, the last known naturally occurring case of smallpox was reported in Somalia in 1977. The United States ceased routine smallpox vaccinations in 1972 and, by 1980, the WHO declared smallpox officially eradicated [1,2]. Globally, routine smallpox immunizations were ceased. All stores of the live smallpox virus were destroyed or transferred to two WHO-approved repositories. One is at the Centers for Disease Control and Prevention (CDC) in Atlanta, Georgia. The second is now at the State Research Center for Virology and Biotechnology in Koltsovo, Russia.

E-mail address: snafziger@uabmc.edu

The concept of using the variola virus as a biological weapon is an old one. During the French and Indian Wars (1754–1767), British soldiers distributed blankets that had been used by smallpox victims, with the intent of initiating an epidemic among Native Americans. The mortality rate associated with these outbreaks was as high as 50% in certain tribes. Scholars have also debated the possibility that smallpox was used as a weapon during the Civil War and by the Japanese military during World War II. Further, there are reports of successful efforts by the former Soviet Union in the 1980s to mass produce the variola virus and adapt it for use as a bioweapon in bombs and missiles. Even more frightening are reports that Russian scientists had been seeking to produce more virulent and lethal recombinant strains of the variola virus for use as a bioweapon. In the post cold-war era, many fear that these experimental weapons could fall into the hands of terrorists or militant nations [3].

Mechanism of toxicity

Smallpox is a double-stranded DNA virus, and is a member of the genus orthopoxvirus, family Poxviridae. The poxvirus genome is the largest known viral genome. The virus has a characteristically brick-shaped structure and is about 200 nm in diameter. Poxviruses are unique because they replicate in the cytoplasm—rather than the nucleus—of host cells. Other members of the orthopox genus (monkeypox, vaccinia) can infect and cause cutaneous lesions in humans, but only smallpox is readily transmitted from person to person.

Variola virus is considered a threatening potential biological weapon because of its aerosol infectivity, stability, and ability to inflict high mortality. Smallpox is spread from person to person primarily via airborne particles and direct contact. Contaminated clothing and bed linens have also been shown to spread the virus [4,5]. Infection occurs through direct contact with mucous membranes or through aerosol exposure. Aerosolized smallpox virus can spread widely and infect many people because it has a very low infectious dosage. Affected individuals remain infectious during the late stages of the incubation period, even though they remain asymptomatic. Depending on the climate, corpses of smallpox victims remain infectious for days to months. Thus, transmission of the disease can occur before the victim exhibits any sign of illness and long after they have died of the disease. The duration of the disease is long and requires complex isolation, which would consume the efforts of many medical personnel and supplies. Finally, there are limited military and no civilian smallpox vaccination requirements at this time, leaving a large susceptible population at risk for smallpox infection.

The reintroduction of smallpox would no doubt lead to deadly epidemics. During the 1960s and 1970s in Europe, as many as 10 to 20 second-generation cases were reported as infected from a single case [1,6]. During the 20th century, smallpox infection was associated with a 1% mortality rate in the vaccinated population and a 30% mortality rate in the unvaccinated population [1]. Because there have not been any large outbreaks of smallpox in many years, it is impossible to predict just what the effect of a large outbreak would be under current circumstances and using current medical technology.

Clinical presentation

The clinical course of smallpox can be thought of in three distinctive phases: incubation, prodromal illness, and overt illness. When inhaled, variola virus travels from the respiratory tract where it attaches to the epithelial cells and replicates. This point is considered the incubation period. The patient is highly infectious because of the high concentration of viral particles replicating in the upper respiratory tract, but remains asymptomatic. The virus is generally transmitted to others through coughing: virus particles are suspended in oropharyngeal secretions.

After an incubation period of 7–14 days following initial exposure, the resulting viremia causes a prodromal illness characterized by high fever, malaise, vomiting, headache, and myalgias. The onset of this high fever marks the end of the incubation period and the beginning of the prodromal illness. During this time, the patient remains highly infectious. Two to three days thereafter, victims will manifest overt smallpox illness, developing a characteristic macular rash about the face, hands, and forearms. As the rash spreads across the body, the macules develop further to papules and eventually to pustular vesicles (Fig. 1). Lesions are most prominent about the extremities and face and tend to develop synchronously. Within 7 to 10 days, the rash begins to form scabs, leaving depressed pigmented scars when they heal. Scabs contain readily recoverable virus throughout the entire healing period; therefore, all patients should be considered infectious until all scabs are shed [7].

Although at least 90% of smallpox cases are clinically characteristic, two other clinical manifestations of smallpox exist and may be difficult to recognize.

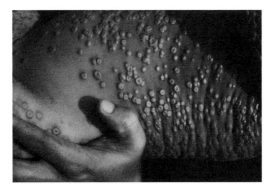

Fig. 1. Typical smallpox lesions.

In fewer than 3% of patients, a "hemorrhagic" form of smallpox will manifest with intense systemic toxicity and mucosal hemorrhage. Five percent of patients will develop "malignant" smallpox, which is characterized by severe systemic toxicity and macular skin lesions. Both of these rare forms of smallpox are associated with very high mortality rates.

Smallpox is most frequently mistaken for varicella, or chickenpox, infection. The most effective criteria for distinguishing the two infections, is an examination of the following characteristics of the skin lesions.

- Time and pattern of appearance. The lesions of chickenpox occur in successive outbreaks (asynchronously). When examining a patient with chickenpox, it is possible to observe skin lesions at several different stages of maturation and development at the same time. In smallpox infection, the skin lesions appear more or less simultaneously (synchronously) and all appear at the same general stage of maturation and development.
- Density and location. Chickenpox lesions tend to be denser over the trunk (centripetal distribution); smallpox lesions are denser on the face and extremities (centrifugal distribution). Chickenpox lesions are almost never seen on the palms or soles of the feet. Smallpox lesions, especially in severe cases, can often be found in these areas.
- Depth and appearance. Chickenpox lesions tend to be superficial vesicles; smallpox lesions are deep-seated and firm, leaving pitted, pigmented scars.

Monkeypox is another consideration in the differential diagnosis of smallpox infection. Patients with monkeypox develop fever, respiratory symptoms, and synchronized lesions like patients with smallpox; however, patients with monkeypox, seem more prone to develop inguinal and cervical lymphadenopathy and appear to have a lower mortality rate (3%–10%). Pneumonia secondary to monkeypox has a 50% mortality rate.

Other common conditions that might be confused with smallpox include disseminated herpes zoster, impetigo, drug eruptions, contact dermatitis, erythema multiforme major and minor, enteroviral infection, scabies, insect bites, and molluscum contagiosum.

Infection control

Because the discovery of even a single case of smallpox would be considered an international health emergency, it is imperative to involve public health officials early when the diagnosis of smallpox is suspected. If a case of smallpox is suspected, the patient must be immediately placed in negative pressure isolation and held, even if against their will, until appropriate assessment is completed by public health authorities. When a case of smallpox is confirmed, all household and face-to-face contacts should be vaccinated and placed under surveillance. Because smallpox is rapidly spread via aerosol transmission, it poses a particular threat in hospitals that have a limited number of negative pressure isolation facilities. Given the serious nature of this disease and the lack of any definitive therapy, home care and quarantine is a likely and reasonable alternative to in-patient hospital treatment for exposed individuals, and may be required with patients able to tolerate oral rehydration in the setting of multiple-victim scenarios.

A post-exposure vaccination program combined with strict quarantine and respiratory isolation should be applied for 17 days to all personnel in direct contact with the index case or cases. This is especially true for all unvaccinated contacts.

Diagnostic studies

There is no widely available laboratory test or other screening tool to confirm smallpox infection; therefore, clinical presentation is the key to early diagnosis. The presence of a centrifugal, synchronous rash in the appropriate clinical setting must lead to consideration of a diagnosis of smallpox.

When a case of smallpox is suspected, definitive laboratory confirmation should be sought as early as possible. State or local health department laboratories should immediately be contacted regarding the collection and shipping of specimens. Someone who has recently been vaccinated (or is vaccinated that day) and who wears gloves and a mask must collect the specimens. To obtain vesicular or pustular fluid, it is often necessary to open lesions with the blunt edge of a scalpel. The fluid can then be harvested on a cotton swab. Scabs can be picked off with forceps. Specimens should be deposited in a sterile vacutainer tube that should be sealed with adhesive tape at the juncture of stopper and tube. This tube, in turn, should be enclosed in a second durable, watertight container.

Laboratory examination and diagnosis requires high-containment (Biosafety Level-4) facilities and should be undertaken only in designated laboratories where appropriate training and equipment is available. In these Biosafety Level-4 laboratories, the presence of smallpox virions can be rapidly confirmed by electron microscopic examination of vesicular or pustular liquid or scabs. Further diagnostic techniques, which use cell cultures and nucleic acid, can also be used to identify variola virus.

Medications and vaccinations

Although animal trials with cidofovir are optimistic, there is currently no treatment for smallpox [8]. There are no data to suggest that cidofovir is more effective than post-exposure vaccination, and the serious renal toxicity of this intravenously administered medication limits its use.

Smallpox vaccine is approved by the US Food and Drug Administration (FDA). The current vaccine supply, which contains live vaccinia virus derived from calves (Dryvax; Wyeth Laboratories, Marietta, Pennsylvania), was created before 1982 and is under the control of the CDC. Recent studies show that dilution of the vaccine by as much as 1:10 is still effective in inducing an appropriate immune response [9,10]. Efforts are underway to increase the national stockpile of smallpox vaccine.

In the past, vaccination has been successfully administered to persons of all ages, from birth onward. Because the vaccine is a live virus, it does have adverse effects associated with its use, including flu-like illness, self-inoculation with appearance of satellite lesions, disseminated rash known as vaccinia, encephalitis, peri-myocarditis, and death in 1 person per 1 million people vaccinated [11]. Because of these risks, vaccination is currently not recommended for certain groups including infants and children, pregnant or breastfeeding women, patients with compromised immune systems, patients with known heart disease, and patients with a history of eczema or other extensive skin diseases, because of the risk of complications. Under epidemic circumstances, however, such contraindications would have to be weighed against the grave risk posed by smallpox. A limited emergency supply of vaccina immune globulin (VIG) is also under the control of the CDC and can be administered concomitantly with vaccination to minimize the risk of complications in these persons [12].

An emergency vaccination program is currently the best way to treat smallpox exposures. Vaccination administered within 4 days of first exposure has been shown to offer some protection against acquiring infection and significant protection against a fatal outcome. An emergency vaccination response would include potentially exposed individuals; all health care workers at facilities that might receive patients; essential disaster response personnel, such as police, firefighters, transit workers, public health staff, and emergency management staff; and mortuary staff who might have to handle bodies. In the event of a smallpox outbreak, it is recommended that all such personnel for whom vaccination is not contraindicated should be vaccinated immediately regardless of prior vaccination status.

In 2003, limited vaccination of health care workers, emergency response personnel, and select military personnel was undertaken in the United States with variable participation. The CDC reports that almost 40,000 civilians were voluntarily vaccinated as part of this effort [13]. It is thought that those who were immunized before 1972 may have partial immunity to smallpox, but the amount of protection related to remote vaccination has not been quantified.

Supportive care

Supportive care for patients with smallpox is limited not only by lack of effective medications, but also by the logistics associated with quarantine or respiratory isolation. Availability of personnel to care for patients can be expected to be a significant limitation. It is not known what percentage of patients infected with smallpox would require advanced intensive care unit therapy such as pressor drugs or ventilatory support. Perhaps with modern medical technology, mortality rates might be less than the historical 30%, but in epidemic situations medical resources would be quickly expended.

Nonetheless, supportive therapy with antibiotics is indicated for treatment of secondary bacterial infections associated with smallpox. Standard supportive care with nutritional and intravenous fluid support should be initiated in those patients who exhibit poor oral intake. Patients with respiratory failure should be assisted with mechanical ventilation as needed.

In an epidemic setting, the institution of home quarantine and provision of limited supportive care in the home or in pre-designated "smallpox hospitals" should be considered because of the extremely infectious nature of this disease.

Clinical course and prognostic factors

Aside from skin lesions, other organs are seldom involved in smallpox infection. Secondary bacterial infection is uncommon. When death does occur, it is usually during the second week of the illness and is thought to be caused by a sepsis-type syndrome. Typically, neutralizing antibodies are present by the sixth day of the rash, which coincides with the onset of clinical improvement. Patients are no longer considered infectious when all scabs have fallen off, which occurs around 21 days after onset of the rash. Survivors may have significant scarring, but exhibit immunity from further infection and typically have no other long-term sequelae [14].

References

[1] Fenner F, Henderson DA, Arita I, et al. Smallpox and its eradication. Geneva, Switzerland: World Health Organization; 1988. p. 1341.

[2] Arita I. Virological evidence for the success of the smallpox eradication programme. Nature 1979;279:293–8.

[3] Alibek K, Handelman S. Biohazard. New York: Dell Publishing; 1999.

[4] Rao AR. Infected inanimate objects and their role in transmission of smallpox. Geneva, Switzerland: World Health Organization; 1972.

[5] Dixon CW. Smallpox. London: J & A Churchill Ltd; 1962. p. 1460.

[6] Wehrle PF, Posch J, Richter KH, et al. An airborne outbreak of smallpox in a German hospital and its significance with respect to other recent outbreaks in Europe. Bull World Health Organ 1970;43:669–79.

[7] Mitra AC, Sarkar JK, Mukherjee MK. Virus content of smallpox scabs. Bull World Health Organ 1974;51:106–7.

[8] LeDuc JW, Jahrling PB. Strengthening national preparedness for smallpox: an update. Emerg Infect Dis 2001;7:155–7.

[9] Frey SE, Newman FK, Cruz J, et al. Dose-related effects of smallpox vaccine. N Engl J Med 2002;346(17):1275–80.

[10] Frey SE, Couch RB, Tacket CO, et al. Clinical responses to undiluted and diluted smallpox vaccine. N Engl J Med 2002;346(17):1265–74.

[11] Lane JM, Ruben FL, Neff JM, et al. Complications of smallpox vaccination, 1968: national surveillance in the United States. N Engl J Med 1969;281:1201–8.

[12] Wharton M, Strika RA, Harpaz R, et al. Recommendations for using smallpox vaccine in a pre-event vaccination program. MMWR 2003;52(RR07):1–16.

[13] Smallpox Vaccination Program Status by State. Available at: www.cdc.gov/od/oc/media/spvaccin.htm. Accessed August 9, 2005.

[14] Breman JG, Henderson DA. Diagnosis and management of smallpox. NEJM 2002;346(17):1300–8.

ELSEVIER
SAUNDERS

Crit Care Clin 21 (2005) 747–763

CRITICAL
CARE
CLINICS

Pulmonary Disease from Biological Agents: Anthrax, Plague, Q Fever, and Tularemia

Mohamud Daya, MD, MS*, Yoko Nakamura, MD

*Department of Emergency Medicine, Oregon Health & Science University,
3181 SW Sam Jackson Park Rd Portland, OR 97239-3098, USA*

Anthrax, plague, Q fever, and tularemia are all bacterial agents that represent a bioterrorism risk to public health according to the Centers for Disease Control and Prevention (CDC) [1]. All have been weaponized for delivery by inhalation and can present with pulmonary manifestations that resemble each other as well as other common endemic illnesses. In this article, we review the threat potential, microbiology, pathogenesis, clinical features, diagnosis, and treatment of each of these agents, and we highlight the similarities and differences between their pulmonary presentations.

Anthrax

Bacillus anthracis is an aerobic, gram-positive, spore-forming, non-motile bacillus whose name is derived from the Greek word for coal (*anthrakis*) because of its characteristic black skin lesions. The organism produces spores when its nutrient supply is exhausted and can survive for decades in this form. Anthrax is primarily a zoonosis, which affects herbivores that graze on endospore-contaminated land. Humans are primarily infected by contact with infected animals or animal products such as hides, wool, and hair.

Anthrax is a Category A biological warfare (BW) agent because of its high lethality and perfectly sized (1–2 μm) spores that can be easily aerosolized [1]. It was a key component of the former United States BW program and was used as a

---

* Corresponding author.
E-mail address: dayam@ohsu.edu (M. Daya).

0749-0704/05/$ – see front matter © 2005 Elsevier Inc. All rights reserved.
doi:10.1016/j.ccc.2005.06.009
criticalcare.theclinics.com

bioweapon by the Japanese army in Manchuria during World War II [2,3]. Although many BW programs were terminated after ratification of the Biological Weapons Convention treaty, some countries secretly continued their programs [3]. In 1979, an outbreak of inhalational anthrax occurred in the Soviet city of Sverdlovsk as a result of an unintentional release of spores from a bioweapons factory [4]. During the 1990s, the extent of the anthrax BW programs in the former Soviet Union and Iraq were discovered and it was learned that the Japanese Aum Shinrikyo cult had released aerosolized anthrax on several occasions [5,6]. In the fall of the 2001, a bioterrorism attack in the United States resulted in 22 cases of anthrax: 11 inhalational and 11 cutaneous. All cases could be linked directly or indirectly (through cross-contamination) by exposure to finely refined *B anthracis* spores, which had been sent in sealed envelopes through the United States Postal Service to selected media outlets and political figures [6,7].

Before the mail contamination attack in 2001, the expected bioterrorism scenario was the delivery of aerosolized anthrax inside a building or over a large outdoor area. An aerial release of *B anthracis* is odorless and invisible and can travel for many kilometers before dispersing [6]. Technology required for large-scale dissemination was developed and tested extensively by the former Soviet Union [5]. A United States government analysis in 1993 estimated that the outdoor release of 100 kg of *B anthracis* upwind of Washington, DC, could produce between 130,000 and 3 million deaths [6].

The major virulence factors of *B anthracis* are plasmid mediated and include its capsule, which allows the vegetative form to resist phagocytosis, and its toxin complex [8]. The latter is composed of 3 proteins: protective antigen, edema factor, and lethal factor. The 3 components combine to form 2 binary toxins: edema toxin and lethal toxin. Protective antigen is common to both toxins and is responsible for attachment to the host cell membrane and subsequent transport into the cell. Edema toxin disrupts water homeostasis by increasing intracellular cylic adenosine monophosphate and is responsible for the massive edema associated with anthrax infections. Lethal toxin is a zinc-dependent protease that leads to death when injected into animals. Its exact mechanism of action remains unclear. Lethal toxin also interferes with the host immune response [9].

Airborne spores greater than 5 μm pose no threat to the lung since they are either filtered in the nasopharynx or cleared by the mucociliary system [6]. Spores that are 1 to 5 μm in size are deposited on the alveolar surface and phagocytosed by alveolar macrophages. Although some spores are lysed, others survive and are transported to mediastinal lymph nodes where they germinate. The factors that trigger germination remain unknown and viable spores have been demonstrated in mediastinal lymph nodes as long as 100 days post-exposure in a rhesus model [6]. In Sverdlovsk, inhalational cases occurred from 2 to 43 days after release of the anthrax spores [4]. Once germination occurs, clinical illness follows rapidly. Initially, extracellular multiplication and local production of the exotoxins leads to mediastinal edema and necrosis. This is followed by systemic bacteremia and toxemia leading to a fulminant death [10]. The median lethal inhalational dose based on animal studies is estimated to be between 2500 to

55,000 spores, but it is likely lower based on the epidemiology of the 2001 attack [6,7].

The classic clinical presentation of inhalation anthrax (IA) is that of a biphasic illness [10]. After an incubation period of 1 to 6 days, the initial stage is characterized by fever, chills, fatigue, minimally productive cough, and chest discomfort. Physical examination is normal and the patient may actually improve transiently. Within 2–3 days, the second stage of the disease develops abruptly with acute dyspnea, fever, profuse diaphoresis, and shock. Massive lympadenopathy and expansion of the mediastinum can lead to subcutaneous edema of the chest and neck with stridor in some cases [10]. Up to half of patients have associated hemorrhagic meningitis with nuchal rigidity, disorientation, and coma. In this stage, cyanosis and hypotension progress rapidly with death within 24–36 hours [10].

Early diagnosis of IA is challenging and requires a high index of suspicion. Routine laboratory tests are not very helpful, although liver function tests may be abnormal in some cases. The most useful screening test is the chest radiograph (Fig. 1A), which may show mediastinal widening, paratracheal fullness, hilar fullness, pleural effusions, and parynchemal infiltrates [11,12]. Abnormalities should be pursued with a chest CT (Fig. 1B) scan, a superior test for demonstrating hemorrhagic lymph nodes, mediastinal edema, and pleural effusions. In the anthrax attacks of 2001, each of the first 10 patients had abnormal chest radiographs, although some findings were subtle: 7 had mediastinal widening, 7 had infiltrates, and 8 had pleural effusions. Each of the 8 patients for whom CT scans were obtained had abnormal results including pleural effusions (8), mediastinal widening (7), and infiltrates (6) [6,12].

During a potential episode of bioterrorism, distinguishing inhalational anthrax from more common disorders such as community-acquired pneumonia (CAP), influenza-like illness (ILI), and other pulmonary BW (Table 1) agents will be

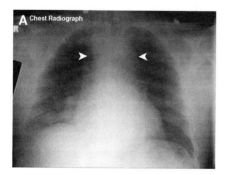
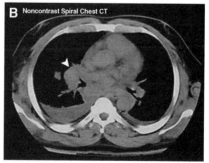

Fig. 1. Portable chest radiograph and non-contrast spiral CT scan of an anthrax patient from 2001. (*A*) Chest radiograph shows a widened mediastinum (*arrowheads*), bilateral hilar fullness, right pleural effusion, and bilateral perihilar airspace disease. (*B*) CT scan shows enlarged right hilar lymph node (*arrowhead*), bilateral pleural effusions, and mediastinal edema. (*From* Mayer TA, Bersoff-Matcha S, Murphy C, et al. Clinical presentation of inhalational anthrax following bioterrorism exposure: report of 2 surviving patients. JAMA 2001;286(20):2549–53; with permission.)

Table 1
Comparison of the microbiological, clinical, radiological and infection control features of the pulmonary BW agents

Features	Anthrax	Plague	Q fever	Tularemia
Biological agent	*Bacillus anthracis*	*Yersinia pestis*	*Coxiella burnetii*	*Francisella tularensis*
Bioterrorism category	A	A	B	A
Bacteriology	Gram-positive bacillus	Gram-negative Coccobacillus Bipolar staining	Gram-negative Pleomorphic rod Intracellular	Gram-negative Coccobacillus Intracellular
Environmental persistence	Yes (spores)	No	Yes (spore-like form)	Yes
Incubation period	1–6 d	2–4 d	14–26 d	3–5 d
Clinical symptoms	Fever, cough, chills, fatigue malaise, lethargy	Fever, productive cough, hemoptysis	Fever, dry cough, pleuritic chest pain, severe headache	Fever, dry cough, malaise, pulse–temperature dissociation
Chest radiograph	Mediastinal widening, pleural effusion, parenchymal infiltrates	Bilateral infiltrates or consolidation, ARDS, cavitation	Segmental and lobar infiltrates, multiple round infiltrates	Segmental or lobar infiltrates, hilar adenopathy, pleural effusions
Chest CT	Hyperdense hilar and mediastinal nodes, infiltrates, pleural effusion	Consolidation, ARDS	Segmental, patchy, or lobar consolidation with or without pleural effusion	Hilar nodes, cavitary lesions
Laboratory studies	WBC count →, Liver enzyme ↑, Hypoxemia	WBC count ↑, Leukemoid reaction	WBC count →, Lymphocyte count ↓, Platelet count ↓, Liver enzyme ↑	WBC ↑, Liver enzyme ↑
Person-to-person transmission	No	Yes	No	No
Precautions	Standard barrier isolation	Respiratory droplet	Standard universal	Standard universal
Respiratory isolation	No	Yes	No	No
Biosafety level	2	2–3	2–3	2–3
Fatality rate	High (fatal if untreated)	High (fatal if untreated)	Low	Moderate

Abbreviation: ARDS, acute respiratory distress syndrome.

challenging. Important clues are patients who suddenly present with severe acute febrile illness and a very fulminant clinical course, or acute febrile illness in association with environmental risk (eg, occupational exposure or epidemiological link to a bioterrorism attack). When compared with ILI in a recent study, the IA patients in 2001 were more likely to have tachycardia, high hematocrit, low sodium, and low albumin, and were less likely to have myalgias, headache, and nasal symptoms [13]. When comparing patients with IA and patients with CAP, IA patients were more likely to have nausea or vomiting, tachycardia, high transaminase levels, low sodium levels, and normal white blood cells counts [13]. In a another article that compared 47 historical cases of inhalational anthrax to 376 controls with CAP or an ILI, the most accurate predictor of inhalation anthrax was the presence of mediastinal widening or pleural effusion on the chest radiograph [14]. This finding was 100% sensitive for IA, 72% specific when compared with CAP, and 96% specific when compared with ILI [14].

The most useful microbiologic test for IA is the routine blood culture, which should show growth in 6 to 24 hours. In 2001, blood cultures were positive in all of the eight IA patients who had them drawn before the initiation of antibiotics [12]. Confirmatory tests are best performed through the Laboratory Response Network (LRN), a group of private and public laboratories established by the CDC. Sputum culture and Gram stain are unlikely to have diagnostic value, given the frequent lack of an associated pneumonic process.

B anthracis is highly susceptible to a variety of antibiotics [3]. Although sensitive to penicillin and ampicillin, the presence of inducible β-lactamases has prompted the CDC to advise against the use of either of these drugs alone for therapy of anthrax [7]. In addition, β-lactamases are not concentrated in phagocytes unlike the fluoroquinolones and cyclines [3]. Current recommendations (Table 2) are based on animal studies and there are no clinical trials on which to base these recommendations [7,15]. Initially, multi-drug therapy is recommended based upon the seriousness of the illness, concern for resistant strains, and success with this strategy in 2001. Clindamycin was included in the initial treatment regimen of some 2001 cases because of its ability to prevent toxin production

Table 2
Treatment of inhalational anthrax in adults

Drug	Dose	Route	Frequency	Duration
Ciprofloxacin	400 mg	IV/PO	Every 12 h	60–100 d
Doxycycline[a]	100 mg	IV/PO	Every 12 h	60–100 d
Levofloxacin	500 mg	IV/PO	Every 24 h	60–100 d
Gatifloxacin	400 mg	IV/PO	Every 24 h	60–100 d
Penicillin G[b]	4 million units	IV	Every 4 h	60–100 d
Amoxicillin[b]	1 g	PO	Every 8 h	60–100 d

Initial treatment should be multi-drug to cover for resistance organisms. Switch to oral therapy when patients condition permits.
Abbreviations: IV, intravenous; PO, by mouth.
[a] Some authors recommend an initial loading dose of 200 mg.
[b] Penicillin should not be used as monotherapy due to the presence of inducible β-lactamases.

in streptococcal disease [11]. Treatment should be continued for 60 days and perhaps as long as 100 days since spores are not affected by antimicrobial therapy [6,7].

Aggressive supportive care is imperative in all cases. Corticosteroids are recommended in patients with extensive edema, respiratory failure, and meningitis [6]. The drainage of pleural fluid, which are typically hemorrhagic, with thoracostomy tubes, reduces the toxin burden in the body and can lead to dramatic clinical improvement [16]. Unfortunately, once toxin production has a reached a threshold level, death occurs in animals even if sterility of the blood is achieved with antibiotics. In Sverdlovsk, the Case Fatality Rate was 86% and in 2001 it was 45%.

Standard universal precautions should be used when caring for patients with all forms of anthrax. Respiratory isolation is not necessary since airborne transmission of anthrax does not occur. The hospital microbiology laboratory should be alerted so that specimen processing occurs under Biosafety Level-2 conditions. Disinfectants such as sodium hypochlorite are effective in cleaning environmental surfaces contaminated with infected bodily fluids [5,15].

Plague

Plague is caused by *Yersinia pestis*, a gram-negative non-spore coccobacillus of the Enterobacteriaceae family [17,18]. Plague is a flea-borne zoonosis, which primarily affects wild and domestic rodents. Other animal hosts include prairie dogs, squirrels, rabbits, chipmunks, and domestic cats. Humans acquire the disease through incidental exposure to infective fleas or through direct contact with infectious tissues and secretions of infected animals or humans [19,20].

Plague is a Category A agent because of its high case fatality rate and potential for human-to-human spread [1]. One of the earliest recorded attempts of BW occurred in 1346 during the siege of Caffa, a coastal town near the Black Sea [2]. The Tartars used catapults to lob corpses of plague victims from their own army into the city with the hope of spreading disease among the Genoese. The attempt was successful, although it is likely that the disease was actually spread by dying rats whose fleas had already left in search of alternate hosts. During World War II, Japan's Unit 731 dropped plague-infected fleas over populated areas of China, which led to outbreaks of plague [21]. Subsequently, BW programs in the United States and the Soviet Union developed techniques to aerosolize plague, thereby eliminating the need for fleas. In the 1990s it was discovered that both Iraq and the former Soviet Union had produced large quantities of dried antibiotic-resistant plague for bombs and missiles [5].

An intentional bioterrorism-related outbreak of plague would most likely occur via an aerosol of the plague bacillus. A plague aerosol is odorless, colorless, and tasteless, and bacteria remain viable for up to 1 hour over a distance of 10 km [21]. In 1970, the World Health Organization (WHO) estimated that a

50 kg release of *Y pestis* over a city of 5 million would initially result in 150,000 cases of pneumonic plague and 36,000 deaths [21].

The virulence of *Y pestis* is based on several factors, many of which are plasmid mediated [17,18,22]. These include the F1, V, and W antigens, which are anti-phagocytic, and plasminogen-activating factor. Also important is the cell-wall-derived lipopolysaccharide endotoxin, which is primarily responsible for the systemic inflammatory response syndrome, which leads to shock, acute respiratory distress syndrome (ARDS), disseminated intravascular coagulation (DIC), and multiple organ failure [22].

Clinical plague has three classical forms, depending on whether the infection enters the lymph nodes (bubonic), the bloodstream (septicemic), or the lungs (pneumonic). Less common presentations include pharyngitis and meningitis [18,22]. Primary pneumonic plague, the most fulminant and fatal form of plague, results from inhaling the aerosolized bacillus. Following an incubation period of 2–4 days, the patient presents with a sudden onset of chills, fever, headache, body pains, weakness, and chest discomfort. In some cases, gastrointestinal symptoms such as abdominal pain and vomiting may also be present. Within 24 hours, there is cough, sputum production, increasing chest pain, tachypnea, and dyspnea. The sputum is most often watery or mucoid, frothy, and blood-tinged, but may become frankly bloody [22]. Chest signs may indicate localized pulmonary involvement with segmental consolidation in the early stage, before the process rapidly spreads to other segments and lobes of the same and opposite lung. The terminal stages are accompanied by hemorrhagic necrosis, acute respiratory failure, and sepsis syndrome with circulatory collapse. Patients with inhalational exposure could also potentially present with pharyngeal plague accompanied by cervical buboes [18].

The early diagnosis of plague requires a high index of suspicion. The sudden onset of a fatal disease in domestic animals, or the appearance of several previously healthy patients with a rapidly progressing pneumonia, suggests the possibility of pneumonic plague especially if there is associated hemoptysis [18,21]. The differential diagnosis includes other causes of severe pneumonia such as Hantavirus pulmonary syndrome, tularemia, and legionnaire's disease. The white blood cell count (WBC) is almost always elevated with a left shift as well as band forms, Dohle bodies, and toxic granulation [18,20,22]. Coagulation abnormalities consistent with DIC are common. Chest radiographs (Fig. 2) show alveolar infiltrates or lobar pneumonia that quickly progresses to diffuse bilateral pneumonitis and ARDS. Microbiologic studies are very valuable in the diagnosis of pneumonic plague. A Gram stain of the sputum may demonstrate the gram-negative bipolar staining organism (closed safety-pin-like appearance) and the bacillus may also be seen in peripheral blood smears [17]. Cultures of sputum or blood will demonstrate growth within 48 hours. A rapid diagnostic test based on the F1 antigen has been developed and field tested in Madagascar [23]. This dipstick test, which is very sensitive and specific, and takes only 15 minutes, can be performed on sputum or serum at the patient's bedside, but is not yet widely available [24]. Confirmatory tests, which include serology, immunostaining, and

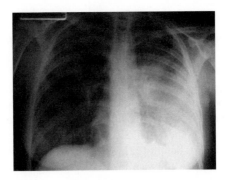

Fig. 2. Chest radiograph of a patient with primary pneumonic plague showing extensive lobar consolidation in the left lower and left middle lung fields. (*From* Inglesby TV, Dennis DT, Henderson DA, et al. Plague as a biological weapon: medical and public health management. JAMA 2000; 283(17):2281–90; with permission.)

polymerase chain reaction (PCR), are available only at specialized laboratories through the LRN. The laboratory should be alerted so that samples are processed under Biosafety Level-2 or -3 conditions.

In the absence of prompt antibiotic treatment (within 24 hours of symptom onset), primary pneumonic plague is almost always fatal [22]. Current treatment recommendations are summarized in Table 3 [16,21]. Penicillin, cephalosporin, and macrolides are ineffective against *Y pestis* and should not be used. Antimicrobial resistance is a concern and multi-drug therapy should be administered initially until sensitivities have been determined [5,25]. Good supportive care, including volume resuscitation and management of the sepsis syndrome with ventilatory support, is imperative [21,22]. Most patients will improve within 2–3 days of beginning treatment and can be switched to oral therapy.

Since pneumonic plague is easily transmitted from person to person, the immediate application of control measures can prevent an epidemic [19]. Although some authors recommend negative pressure rooms and class N95 respirators,

Table 3
Treatment recommendations for adults with pneumonic plague

Drug	Dose	Route	Frequency	Duration
Streptomycin	1 g	IM	Every 12 h	10 d
Gentamicin	5 mg/kg	IM, IV	Every 24 h	10 d
Gentamicin	1.75 mg/kg	IV	Every 8 h	10 d
Ciprofloxacin	400 mg	IV/PO	Every 12 h	10 d
Levofloxacin	500 mg	IV/PO	Every 24 h	10 d
Gatifloxacin	400 mg	IV/PO	Every 24 h	10 d
Doxycycline[a]	100 mg	IV/PO	Every 12 h	14 d
Tetracycline	500 mg	PO	Every 6 h	14 d

Switch to oral therapy when patient's condition has improved.
Abbreviations: IM, intramuscular; IV, intravenous; PO, by mouth.
    [a] Some authors recommend an initial loading dose of 200 mg.

there is no epidemiological evidence that plague can be spread from person to person by droplet nuclei (< 5 μm) [18,26]. Patients should be cared for using contact and respiratory isolation to prevent droplet (> 5 μm) spread [21,26]. This can be accomplished using surgical masks, gown, gloves, and eye protection [21]. Patients being transported should also wear surgical masks [21]. Contaminated bedding and clothing of patients can be disinfected according to hospital protocol. Environmental decontamination of an area exposed to a plague aerosol is unnecessary because the vegetative organism does not survive for long outside a host [17,21].

Q fever

Q (query) fever is a worldwide zoonosis caused by the bacterium *Coxiella burnetii*, which can lead to acute and occasionally chronic infection in humans. Common animal reservoirs are domesticated ruminants such as cattle, sheep, and goats. Humans usually acquire Q fever by inhaling aerosols or contaminated dusts derived from infected animals or animal products. Derrick first described Q fever in 1937 while investigating an undiagnosed febrile illness in abattoir workers in Brisbane, Queensland [27].

C burnetii is a small (0.2 × 0.7 μm) obligate intracellular gram-negative bacterium whose spore-like form can survive for months or years in harsh environments [28,29]. It has been mass-produced and weaponized by several biological warfare programs [5,30]. Although it is unclear if Q fever has ever been used as a biological weapon, outbreaks were reported during World War II and more recently during the Balkan conflict [31]. Most of these epidemics were subsequently attributed to inhalation of naturally occurring dust-borne *C burnetii*. In 1987, an outbreak of Q fever affected postmen in Oxfordshire, United Kingdom. Although the source was never found, contamination of mail from rural areas was suspected to have transported *C burnetii* into the post office [32].

Its widespread availability, high infectivity (infective dose is 1–10 organisms), consistent ability to cause disability, potential for mass production, environmental persistence, ease of aerosol dissemination, and limited vaccine availability make it an ideal biological warfare agent [31,33]. Q fever is classified as a Category B agent since it lacks the capacity to cause mass fatalities [1]. *C burnetii* could be used as a debilitating biological weapon in an aerosolized form or as a contaminant of food, water, or possibly mail [31].

Following inhalation or ingestion, *C burnetii* attach to host macrophages by way of spectrin-binding proteins called ankyrins, and the bacterium is internalized. These phagosomes then fuse with lysosomes to form phagolysosomes [28]. *C burnetii* has cleverly adapted itself to survive, multiply, and disseminate within the hostile environment of the acidic phagolysosome. Although both humoral and cell mediated immunity (CMI) are important in controlling *C burnetii*, the latter appears to be more important. Impaired CMI (pregnancy, immunosupression) is an established risk factor for chronic infection. Immunity to Q fever is non-sterile and the organism persists in the host and can cause relapse of the disease [31].

Release of the aerosolized form of Coxiella in a densely populated area would cause the abrupt onset of illness similar to that seen with the naturally occurring disease. Up to 60% of naturally occurring infections are asymptomatic. Symptomatic illness can be divided into acute and chronic forms. After an incubation period of 14 to 26 days (dependent on the inoculum dose), the disease can present as a self-limited flu-like illness, pneumonia, or hepatitis [28]. Clinical presentation depends on the route of infection as well as host factors [28,29]. Less common acute presentations include pericarditis, myocarditis, and meningo-encephalitis [34]. The flu-like syndrome lasts 1–3 weeks and is characterized by the sudden onset of high fever, diaphoresis, headache, and myalgias. Although symptoms resolve, general malaise may persist for months. Most cases of Q fever pneumonia are mild and present with fever, retro-orbital headache, non-productive cough, and pleuritic chest pain. The headache can be very severe and is more common then in CAP associated with other organisms [29]. Crackles can be auscultated in 50% of cases and only 2% of patients will have respiratory distress severe enough to require ICU admission [29]. Hepatitis can be symptomatic or clinically silent and manifested only by biochemical abnormalities [34]. Chronic Q fever is defined as infection lasting for more than 6 months [28]. It occurs in approximately 1% of patients infected with *C burnetii* and the classic presentation is that of endocarditis involving abnormal or prosthetic cardiac valves.

The initial picture of acute Q fever will be difficult to differentiate clinically from a naturally occurring outbreak of influenza or other causes of atypical pneumonia, such as Mycoplasma, Chlamydia, Legionella, or various viruses. In addition, other bioterrorism agents that cause influenza-like illnesses such as plague, anthrax, and tularemia, must also be considered (see Table 1). Glanders and brucellosis are also considerations in patients with abrupt fever, headache, and myalgias [31]. If 50 kg of *C burnetii* was released along a 2 km line upwind of a population of 500,000, it has been estimated that there would be 150 deaths, 125,000 cases of acute illness, and 9000 cases of chronic illness. Panic and fear would cause many additional illnesses [31].

The clinical, laboratory, and radiological findings of acute Q fever are non-specific and the diagnosis is best made through serology. The leukocyte count is usually normal but lymphopenia is common and thrombocytopenia is noted in 25% of cases [29]. Liver enzymes are elevated in as many as 85% of cases. Prolonged fever with a normal WBC count, thrombocytopenia, and elevated hepatic enzymes should prompt the consideration of Q fever. The most common abnormalities on chest radiography are segmental or lobar opacities [35]. Pleural effusions are seen in only 10% of patients and mediastinal lympadenopathy is uncommon. Although uncommon, multiple rounded opacities (Fig. 3) are a hallmark of Q fever pneumonia [29]. The typical finding on chest CT is multilobar airspace consolidation [36].

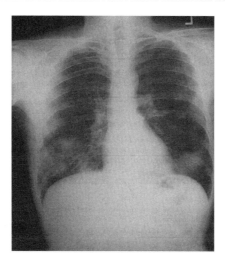

Fig. 3. Chest radiograph of a young man with Q fever pneumonia and multiple rounded opacities. The patient was exposed to an infected parturient cat. (*From* Marrie T. Q Fever. In: Guerrant RL, Walker DH, Weller PF, editors. Tropical infectious diseases: principles, pathogens, and practice, Volume 1. Philadelphia: Churchill Livingstone; 1999; with permission.)

An immunofluorescence assay is the current reference method for the sero-diagnosis of Q fever [28]. Approximately 90% of patients have detectable antibodies by the third week [28]. In acute Q fever, IgM and IgG titers to phase II antigens are higher then that to phase I antigens, and in chronic Q fever, the reverse is true. More rapid or novel diagnostic tests such as ELISA or PCR may be useful in a bioterrorism event.

Q fever is a usually a self-limited disease that resolves spontaneously within 2 weeks and the case fatality rate is less then 1% [34]. The recommended anti-

Table 4
Treatment recommendations for adults with coxiella pneumonia

Drug	Dose	Route	Frequency	Duration
Doxycycline[a]	100 mg	IV/PO	Every 12 h	14 d
Tetracycline	500 mg	PO	Every 6 h	14 d
Ofloxacin	200 mg	PO	Every 8 h	14 d
Pefloxacin	400 mg	PO/IV	Every 12 h	14 d
Erythromycin[b]	500 mg	PO	Every 6 h	14 d
Azithromycin	500 mg loading dose, then 250 mg	PO/IV	Every 24 h	5 d
Clarithromycin	500 mg	PO	Every 12 h	14 d

Begin with parenteral therapy in severe cases and switch to oral regimen based on clinical response. *Abbreviations:* IV, intravenous; PO, by mouth.

[a] For patients with underlying valvular heart disease, treatment should be extended to one year in conjunction with hydroxycholorquine to prevent Q fever endocarditis.

[b] Not recommended in severe cases and use is controversial because in vitro resistance and treatment failures have been reported.

biotic treatment options for acute Q fever pneumonia are summarized in Table 4 [29,31,34]. In general, the cyclines, fluoroquinolones, and macrolides are effective against *C burnetti*. Treatment is most effective if initiated early. Because of the risk of chronic infection, clinical and serological follow-up for 1 year is recommended.

Person-to-person transmission is rare and respiratory isolation is not required [29]. Standard universal precautions should be followed and solutions of sodium hypochlorite (0.5%), phenol (1%), or hydrogen peroxide (5%) can be used for environmental decontamination [31]. Biosafety Level-2 or -3 precautions should be followed when processing tissue samples and when dealing with pregnant patients.

Tularemia

Tularemia is a zoonosis of lagomorphs and rodents caused by *Francisella tularensis*, an intracellular aerobic gram-negative coccobacillus. *F tularensis* does not form spores but can survive for weeks under adverse conditions in water, moist soil, animal carcasses, hay, and straw [37,38]. Of the known subspecies, the most virulent for humans is *F tularensis tularensis* (Group A) [39]. Infection with *F tularensis holoartica* (Group B) results in a milder nonfatal illness [39]. The disease is transmitted to humans through the handling of infected animals; bites of arthropod vectors such as ticks, deerflies, fleas, and mosquitoes; ingestion of contaminated food, water, or soil; and inhalation of infective aerosols [38,40,41]. A recent outbreak (Group A) on Martha's Vineyard was attributed to infective aerosols generated by lawn mowing and brush cutting [42].

F tularensis is a Category A agent because of its high infectivity (inhalation or inoculation of as few as 50 organisms can cause disease), ease of dissemination, and ability to cause substantial illness and death [1,38]. It was studied extensively by the Japanese during their World War II occupation of Manchuria and was weaponized and stockpiled by the United States military [2,37,38]. The former Soviet Union also maintained stockpiles that included strains, which were resistant to antibiotics and vaccines [2,4,38]. It is unclear if tularemia has ever been used for biological warfare. In his book *Biohazard*, former Soviet expert Dr. Ken Alibek alleged that Russia used tularemia against German troops during the battle for Stalingrad in 1942 [5]. A recent review, however, proposes that a naturally occurring outbreak, facilitated by conditions of war, was a more likely explanation for the epidemic [43].

Although *F tularensis* could be used as a weapon in a number of ways, the most concerning scenario is that of an aerosol release. Modeling studies conducted by the WHO in 1970 estimated that an aerosol dispersal of 50 kg of virulent *F tularensis* over a metropolitan area with 5 million inhabitants would result in 250,000 incapacitating casualties, including 19,000 deaths [38]. Symptoms would persist for several weeks and disease relapses would occur for many months. In addition, such a release might lead to the establishment of enzootic reservoirs of tularemia in wild animals, which would result in subsequent outbreaks of human disease [39].

The virulence factors of F tularensis are not well understood. F tularensis is a facultative intracellular bacterium whose primary target is the macrophage [39]. The bacteria enter the macrophage through phagosomes and are able to avoid the normally lethal respiratory burst. They subsequently escape into the cytoplasm and begin to proliferate. The macrophage then undergoes apoptosis releasing large numbers of bacteria that can infect new cells [39]. Other known virulence factors are a capsule and cell wall lipopolysaccharide, although the latter does not behave like a typical endotoxin [39]. In addition to local multiplication, involvement of regional lymph nodes and systemic bacteremia is common. The initial tissue reaction to infection is a focal, intensely suppurative necrosis, which consists largely of accumulations of polymorphonuclear leukocytes, followed by invasion of macrophages, epithelioid cells, and lymphocytes [38]. Suppurative lesions are eventually transformed into granulomatous lesions with a central necrotic zone [38]. Like many other intracellular organisms, humoral immunity is less protective and it is the presence of cell-mediated immunity that ultimately controls and contains the infection [44].

After an incubation period of 1 to 21 days (average 3–5 days), early infection is characterized by abrupt onset of fever, chills, myalgias, arthralgias, and fatigue. Pulse–temperature dissociation is often noted [44,45]. Depending on the route of infection, F tularensis can result in one of six clinical syndromes: ulceroglandular, glandular, oculoglandular, oropharyngeal, typhoidal, and pneumonic [38,40,44]. These syndromes are not distinct and overlapping features are common. All can result in hematogenous spread leading to meningitis, pericarditis, hepatitis, endocarditis, osteomyelitis, sepsis syndrome, rhabdomyolysis, and acute renal failure [38,40]. Lung involvement is caused by either hematogenous (secondary pneumonia) or airborne spread. Primary pneumonic tularemia is the most severe clinical form of tularemia; the mortality rate is as high as 60% in the absence of treatment [41]. The initial presentation is that of a systemic illness without prominent signs of respiratory disease, although there may be dry cough and pleuritic chest pain. The patient will eventually develop signs and symptoms of typical bronchopneumonia often involving more than one lobe. Rarely, pulmonary infection can lead to severe pneumonia, ARDS, and death [38].

The diagnosis of pneumonic tularemia is challenging and requires a high index of suspicion. The presence of a cluster of acute atypical pneumonia with unusual epidemiological features and lack of response to conventional therapy should lead clinicians to consider tularemia. The differential diagnosis of pneumonic tularemia includes other causes of atypical pneumonia such as Mycoplasma, Chlamydia, Legionella, as well as other pulmonary BW agents (see Table 1). The clinical course of pneumonic tularemia is usually less fulminant then that seen with IA or plague [38].

The laboratory diagnosis of tularemia is also very challenging. Nonspecific findings include a leukocytosis and abnormal liver enzyme levels in 50% of cases. Chest radiograph findings in one series consisted of patchy unilateral or

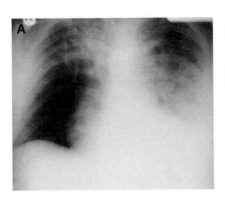
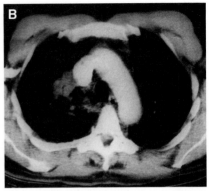

Fig. 4. Chest radiograph and contrast spiral CT scan of a tularemia patient. (*A*) Chest radiograph shows extensive consolidation of the left lung field and a moderate left pleural effusion. (*B*) CT scan of the chest shows a nodular opacity in the right upper lobe with air bronchograms. (*From* Shapiro DS, Mark EJ. Case 14-2000— A 60-year-old farm worker with bilateral pneumonia. NEJM 2002; 342(19):1430–8; with permission.)

bilateral subsegmental air space opacities (74%), hilar lymphadenopathy (32%), and pleural effusion (30%) [46]. Additional features include cavitary lesions, many of which may be better visualized on a chest CT scan (Fig. 4) [45,46]. Cultures of sputum, blood, and other body fluids are frequently negative because the organism is very fastidious and requires cysteine for growth [37,38,41]. Communication with the laboratory is essential so that growth conditions can be optimized. Advanced methods such as antigen detection and PCR, available through the Reference Laboratory Network, can establish the diagnosis more rapidly since serological tests take more then 10 days to attain diagnostic levels [38].

In addition to good supportive care, prompt antibiotic treatment is important for a successful outcome. Current recommendations are summarized in Table 5. Aminoglycosides and the fluoroquinolones are therapies of choice in severely ill

Table 5
Treatment recommendations for adults with tularemia pneumonia

Drug	Dose	Route	Frequency	Duration
Streptomycin	1 g	IM	Every 12 h	10 d
Gentamicin	5 mg/kg	IM, IV	Every 24 h	10 d
Ciprofloxacin	400 mg	IV	Every 12 h	10 d
Levofloxacin	500 mg	IV	Every 24 h	10 d
Gatifloxacin	400 mg	IV	Every 24 h	10 d
Doxycycline	100 mg	IV	Every 12 h	14 d
Tetracycline	500 mg	PO	Every 6 h	14 d
Chloramphenicol	500 mg	IV	Every 6 h	14 d

Begin with parenteral therapy in severe cases and switch to oral regimen based on clinical response.
Abbreviations: IM, intramuscular; IV, intravenous; PO, by mouth.

patients [15,38,40,44]. Relapses are more common with the cyclines and chloramphenicol, although this may be obviated through longer courses of therapy. Macrolides, β-lactams, and lincosamides are ineffective [44].

Standard universal precautions should be followed and respiratory isolation is not necessary since person-to-person transmission has not been reported. Sodium hypochlorite is effective for surface decontamination [15]. *F tularensis* is an occupational hazard for laboratory personnel and specimen handling should be performed under Biosafety Level-2 or -3 conditions depending on the risk for aerosol exposure [38].

Summary

Anthrax, plague, Q fever, and tularemia are all uncommon bacterial infections whose pulmonary manifestations can be readily confused with each other as well as other more common diseases, such as influenza and atypical pneumonia. Each of these agents should be included in the differential diagnosis of a severe or rapidly progressive pneumonic illness. The rapid identification and treatment of potentially affected individuals and the institution of appropriate infection control measures is of primary importance in the public health response to bioterrorism [47].

References

[1] Rotz LD, Khan AS, Lillibridge SR, et al. Public health assessment of potential biological terrorism agents. Emerg Infect Dis 2002;8:225–30.

[2] Jacobs MK. The history of biologic warfare and bioterrorism. Dermatol Clin 2004;22:231–46.

[3] Bryskier A. *Bacillus anthracis* and antibacterial agents. Clin Microbiol Infect 2002;8:467–78.

[4] Abramova FA, Grinberg LM, Yampolskaya OV, et al. Pathology of inhalational anthrax in 42 cases from the Sverdlovsk outbreak of 1979. Proc Natl Acad Sci USA 1993;90:2291–4.

[5] Alibek K, Handleman S. Biohazard: the chilling true story of the largest covert biological weapons program in the world. New York: Random House; 1999.

[6] Inglesby TV, O'Toole T, Henderson DA, et al. Anthrax as a biological weapon, 2002: updated recommendations for management. JAMA 2002;287:2236–52.

[7] Centers for Disease Control and Prevention. Update: investigation of bioterrorism-related anthrax and interim guidelines for exposure management and antimicrobial therapy, October 2001. MMWR 2001;50:909–19.

[8] Mourez M, Lacy DB, Cunningham K, et al. 2001: a year of major advances in anthrax toxin research. Trends Microbiol 2002;10:287–93.

[9] Fukao T. Immune system paralysis by anthrax lethal toxin: the roles of innate and adaptive immunity. Lancet Infect Dis 2004;4:166–70.

[10] Brachman PS. Inhalation anthrax. Ann NY Acad Sci 1980;353:83–93.

[11] Mayer TA, Bersoff-Matcha S, Murphy C, et al. Clinical presentation of inhalational anthrax following bioterrorism exposure: report of 2 surviving patients. JAMA 2001;286:2549–53.

[12] Jernigan JA, Stephens DS, Ashford DA, et al. Bioterrorism-related inhalational anthrax: the first 10 cases reported in the United States. Emerg Infect Dis 2001;7:933–44.

[13] Kuehnert MJ, Doyle TJ, Hill HA, et al. Clinical features that discriminate inhalational anthrax from other acute respiratory illnesses. Clin Infect Dis 2003;36:328–36.

[14] Kyriacou DN, Stein AC, Yarnold PR, et al. Clinical predictors of bioterrorism-related inhalational anthrax. Lancet 2004;364:449–52.

[15] Cunha BA. Anthrax, tularemia, plague, ebola or smallpox as agents of bioterrorism: recognition in the emergency room. Clin Microbiol Infect 2002;8:489–503.

[16] Bell DM, Kozarsky PE, Stephens DS. Clinical issues in the prophylaxis, diagnosis, and treatment of anthrax. Emerg Infect Dis 2002;8:222–5.

[17] Perry RD, Fetherston JD. Yersinia pestis – etiologic agent of plague. Clin Microbiol Rev 1997; 10:35–66.

[18] Cobbs CG, Chansolme DH. Plague. Dermatol Clin 2004;22:303–12.

[19] Ratsitorahina M, Chanteau S, Rahalison L, et al. Epidemiological and diagnostic aspects of the outbreak of pneumonic plague in Madagascar. Lancet 2000;355:111–3.

[20] Meyer K. Pneumonic plague. Bacteriol Rev 1961;25:249–61.

[21] Inglesby TV, Dennis DT, Henderson DA, et al. Plague as a biological weapon: medical and public health management. JAMA 2000;283:2281–90.

[22] Dennis DT, Meier FA. Plague. In: Horsburgh Jr CR, Nelson AM, editors. Pathology of emerging infections. Washington (DC): American Society for Microbiology; 1997. p. 21–47.

[23] Chanteau S, Rahalison L, Ralafiarisoa L, et al. Development and testing of a rapid diagnostic test for bubonic and pneumonic plague. Lancet 2003;361:211–6.

[24] Dennis DT, Chu MC. A major new test for plague. Lancet 2003;361:191–2.

[25] Galimand M, Guiyoule A, Gerbaud G, et al. Multidrug resistance in Yersinia pestis mediated by a transferable plasmid. N Engl J Med 1997;337:677–80.

[26] Inglesby TV, Henderson DA, O'Toole T, et al. Safety precautions to limit exposure from plague-infected patients. JAMA 2000;284:1648–9.

[27] Derrick EH. Q fever, a new entity: clinical features, diagnosis and laboratory investigation. Med J Aust 1937;2:281–99.

[28] Maurin M, Raoult D. Q Fever. Clin Microbiol Rev 1999;12:518–33.

[29] Marrie TJ. Coxiella burnetii pneumonia. Eur Respir J 2003;2:713–9.

[30] Seshadri R, Paulsen IT, Eisen JA, et al. Complete genome sequence of the Q-fever pathogen Coxiella burnetii. Proc Natl Acad Sci USA 2003;100:5455–60.

[31] Madariaga MG, Rezai K, Trenholme GM, et al. Q fever: a biological weapon in your backyard. Lancet Infect Dis 2003;2:709–21.

[32] Winner SJ, Eglin RP, Moore VI, et al. An outbreak of Q fever affecting postal workers in Oxfordshire. J Infect 1987;14:255–61.

[33] Cutler SJ, Paiba GA, Howells J, et al. Q fever – a forgotten disease. Lancet Infect Dis 2002; 2:717–8.

[34] Raoult D, Tissot-Dupont H, Foucault C, et al. Q fever 1985–1998: clinical and epidemiological features of 1,383 infections. Medicine 2000;79:109–23.

[35] Gikas A, Kofteridis D, Bouros D, et al. Q fever pneumonia: appearance on chest radiographs. Radiology 1999;210:339–43.

[36] Voloudaki AE, Kofteridis DP, Tritou IN, et al. Q fever pneumonia: CT findings. Radiology 2000;215:800–83.

[37] Cronquist SD. Tularemia: the disease and the weapon. Dermatol Clin 2004;22:313–20.

[38] Dennis DT, Inglesby TV, Henderson DA, et al. Tularemia as a biological weapon: medical and public health management. JAMA 2001;285:2763–73.

[39] Oyston PC, Sjostedt A, Titball RW. Tularemia: bioterrorism defense renews interest in Francisella tularensis. Nat Rev Microbiol 2004;2:967–78.

[40] Choi E. Tularemia and Q fever. Med Clin North Am 2002;86:393–416.

[41] Hornick R. Tularemia revisited. N Engl J Med 2001;345:1637–9.

[42] Feldman KA, Enscore RE, Lathrop SL, et al. An outbreak of primary pneumonic tularemia on Martha's Vineyard. N Engl J Med 2001;345:1601–6.

[43] Croddy E, Krcalova S. Tularemia, biological warfare, and the battle for Stalingrad (1942–1943). Mil Med 2001;166:837–8.

[44] Tarnvik A, Berglund L. Tularemia. Eur Respir J 2003;21:361–73.
[45] Shapiro DS, Mark EJ. Case 14–2000. A 60-year-old farm worker with bilateral pneumonia. N Engl J Med 2000;342:1430–8.
[46] Rubin SA. Radiographic spectrum of pleuropulmonary tularemia. AJR Am J Roentgenol 1978; 131:277–81.
[47] Rotz LD, Hughes JM. Advances in detecting and responding to threats from bioterrorism and emerging infectious disease. Nat Med 2004;10:S130–6.

ELSEVIER
SAUNDERS

CRITICAL
CARE
CLINICS

Crit Care Clin 21 (2005) 765–783

Hemorrhagic Fever Viruses

David C. Pigott, MD

Department of Emergency Medicine, The University of Alabama at Birmingham,
619 South 19ᵗʰ Street, Birmingham, AL 35249-7013, USA

Viral hemorrhagic fevers (VHF) are a group of febrile illnesses caused by RNA viruses from several viral families. They include species from the family of filoviruses (Ebola and Marburg), from the family of arenaviruses (Lassa and New World arenaviruses), from the family of bunyaviruses (Congo-Crimean Hemorrhagic Fever and Rift Valley Fever), and from the family of flaviviruses (yellow fever, among others). These highly infectious viruses lead to a potentially lethal disease syndrome characterized by fever, malaise, vomiting, mucosal and gastrointestinal (GI) bleeding, edema, and hypotension. The most notorious member of this group is the Ebola virus, which has been associated with case fatality rates of up to 90%. These diseases are generally contracted via an infected animal or arthropod vector, although the natural reservoirs for some VHF, such as Ebola and Marburg, remain unknown (Table 1) [1].

In 2000, the Centers for Disease Control and Prevention (CDC) Strategic Planning Workgroup developed a system for categorizing potential agents of bioterrorism into Categories A, B, and C. Those agents in Category A are believed to pose the greatest threat to public health because of ease of dissemination or transmission, potential for high mortality, and significant impact on public health including panic, social, and economic disruption [2]. Along with infectious agents such as anthrax and smallpox, several VHF viruses are classified as Category A: Ebola, Marburg, Lassa, Junin, Machupo, Guanarito, and Sabia. This review will focus on those VHF agents that may represent the greatest threat of bioterrorism, although this should not suggest that other VHF agents could not be used as biological weapons.

The VHF viruses considered to have the greatest potential risk as biological warfare agents share certain characteristics: extreme pathogenicity, and potential

---

Figure Legends (please note: the figures and tables included with this work are from US Government publications and are in the public domain).

E-mail address: dpigott@uabmc.edu

0749-0704/05/$ – see front matter © 2005 Elsevier Inc. All rights reserved.
doi:10.1016/j.ccc.2005.06.007   *criticalcare.theclinics.com*

Table 1
Recognized viral hemorrhagic fevers of humans

Virus **family** genus	Disease (virus)	Natural distribution	Source of human infection		Incubation (days)
			Usual	Less likely	
Arenaviridae					
Arenavirus	Lassa fever	Africa	Rodent	Nosocomial	5–16
	Argentine HF (Junin)	South America	Rodent	Nosocomial	7–14
	Bolivian HF (Machupo)	South America	Rodent	Nosocomial	9–15
	Brazilian HF (Sabia)	South America	Rodent	Nosocomial	7–14
	Venezuelan HF (Guanarito)	South America	Rodent	Nosocomial	7–14
Bunyaviridae					
Phlebovirus	Rift Valley fever	Africa	Mosquito	Slaughter of domestic animal	2–15
Nairovirus	Crimean-Congo HF	Europe, Asia, Africa	Tick	Slaughter of domestic animal; nosocomial	3–12
Hantavirus	HFRS (Hantaan and related viruses)	Asia, Europe; possible worldwide	Rodent		9–35
Filoviridae					
Filovirus	Marburg and Ebola HF	Africa	Unknown	Nosocomial	3–16
Flaviviridae					
Flavivirus					
(Mosquito-borne)	Yellow fever	Tropical Africa, South America	Mosquito		3–6
	Dengue HF	Asia, Americas, Africa	Mosquito		Unknown for dengue HF, but 3–5 for uncomplicated dengue
(Tick-borne)	Kyasanur Forest disease	India	Tick		3–8
	Omsk HF	Soviet Union	Tick	Muskrat-contaminated water	3–8

Abbreviations: HF, hemorrhagic fever; HFRS, hemorrhagic fever with renal syndrome.
Jahrling P. Viral hemorrhagic fevers. In: Textbook of military medicine, Volume 1. Falls Church (VA): Office of the Surgeon General; 1989.

for transmission by fine particle aerosol. The potential for droplet or aerosol spread of these viruses has been largely responsible for intense academic and military interest in these agents. The Working Group on Civilian Biodefense recently published an analysis of the potential of VHF agents for use as a bioterrorist weapon [3]. They emphasize the great infectivity, ease of transmission, risk to public health, and high mortality associated with these infectious agents as reasons for their biological weapon potential.

Hemorrhagic fever viruses have been weaponized by the former Soviet Union and the United States as part of previous biological weapon programs but no confirmed use of these agents has been reported [4]. Dr. Ken Alibek, the former deputy director of the once-massive Soviet bioweapons program, Biopreparat, claims Soviet scientists successfully had produced a stable Marburg virus biological weapon that could be delivered as an aerosol [5]. Hemorrhagic fever viruses have also been of interest to terrorist groups. Aum Shinrikyo, the Japanese religious cult behind the 1995 Tokyo subway sarin gas attacks [6], sent members to Africa in 1992 to obtain samples of Ebola virus for use in a bioweapon, but was unsuccessful in securing the virus [7].

Mechanism of toxicity

The use of VHF agents as a biological weapon has been the subject of avid speculation in the popular media and dramatized in books and film by showing a panicked populace in the throes of a rapidly spreading epidemic. The reality is likely to be far less cinematic, although public perceptions of the risk may lead to significant social and economic disruption. The most likely method for spread of VHF is by fine-droplet aerosol, although contamination of surfaces, food, and water are other potential sources of infection. A terrorist group equipped with a sufficient supply of a highly contagious VHF agent, such as Ebola or Marburg, in an environmentally stable form, could cause a mass casualty event with high morbidity and mortality. Multiple studies in nonhuman primates have documented the aerosol spread of Ebola virus [8–10], and droplet spread has been suspected as a mode of disease transmission among infected humans; although, human-to-human aerosol transmission appears to be rare [11].

Although species in the family of filoviruses, such as Ebola and Marburg, likely represent the greatest bioterrorism threat, other VHF agents are also transmissible by droplet spread. Aerosol transmission of Lassa virus, a species in the genus arenavirus endemic in western Africa, has been documented in nonhuman primates under laboratory conditions [12]. During a 1969 outbreak in Nigeria, an index patient transmitted Lassa to 16 other patients in the same hospital ward; transmission was thought to be by way of droplet aerosol spread [13]. As with Lassa virus infection, some viruses from the family of arenaviruses, such as Junin, are typically acquired by way of aerosolization of infected rodent excreta, particularly urine [14], but laboratory workers working with these agents have been become infected through inhalation of aerosols [15]. Similar laboratory-related aerosol transmission has also been described with yellow fever [16].

The most commonly documented method of filovirus transmission has been by direct contact with blood, body fluids, or tissue of infected persons or nonhuman primates. A recent review of wild animal mortality and human Ebola outbreaks in Gabon and the Republic of Congo concluded that all human Ebola outbreaks in this region from 2001 to 2003 resulted from handling infected wild animal carcasses [17]. Analysis of 21 carcasses revealed that 10 gorillas, 3 chimpanzees, and 1 duiker, a small African deer, were infected with Ebola. The discovery of wild animals infected with Ebola does not establish that these animals are natural filovirus reservoirs. Ebola is rapidly fatal in these animals, suggesting that they are not the natural host [18]. Research into the natural host for Ebola is ongoing, with recent work suggesting that small mammals with little contact with humans, such as bats, may be a natural reservoir for filoviruses such as Ebola and Marburg [19].

During the 2000–2001 Ebola outbreak in Uganda, there were 224 (53%) deaths from 425 presumptive case patients [11]. Three important means of disease transmission were identified during this outbreak: ritual contact with bodies of deceased patients, intrafamilial transmission, and nosocomial spread. In addition, 14 (64%) of 22 of health care workers involved with the care of patients infected with Ebola were also infected, despite the establishment of isolation wards. Once stricter infection control measures were instituted, disease containment was achieved. The ease of person-to-person transmission of Ebola virus is supported by the presence of Ebola virus in the skin and sweat glands of infected persons, as documented by immunohistochemical assay [20].

Conversely, during the 1999 outbreak of Marburg virus infection in Durba, Republic of Congo, few cases of clear person-to-person transmission could be verified [21]. The causative agent behind an ongoing outbreak of hemorrhagic fever in Angola that began in October 2004 was recently identified as Marburg virus. While epidemiologic studies of this outbreak are still underway, it appears that of the 102 identified cases, 95 have died; 75% of deaths were children [22]. The route of transmission of this infection is not yet known, although a small number of health care workers have already been infected. The primary mode of initial arenavirus infection is aerosolized rodent excreta, typically urine, as rodents are the natural reservoirs of the arenaviruses. Person-to-person transmission of arenaviruses such as Lassa is—as with filoviruses—primarily via contact with infected blood and body fluids [14,23].

The primary pathologic defect in patients with VHF is that of increased vascular permeability [24,25]. Hemorrhagic fever viruses have an affinity for the vascular system, leading initially to signs such as flushing, conjunctival injection, and petechial hemorrhages, usually associated with fever and myalgias. Later, frank mucous membrane hemorrhage may occur, with accompanying hypotension, shock, and circulatory collapse. The relative severity of the clinical presentation may vary depending on the virus in question, amount, and route of exposure.

In acute disease, patients are extremely viremic, and messenger RNA (mRNA) evidence of multiple cytokine activation exists [26]. In vitro studies reveal these cytokines lead to shock and increased vascular permeability, the basic pathophysiologic processes most often seen in VHF infection [27]. Another prominent pathologic feature is pronounced macrophage involvement [28]. Inadequate or delayed immune response to these novel viral antigens may lead to rapid development of overwhelming viremia. Extensive infection and necrosis of affected organs also are described. Hemorrhagic complications are multifactorial and are related to hepatic damage, consumptive coagulopathy, and primary marrow injury to megakaryocytes. The increased vascular permeability in VHF infection is thought to be secondary to endothelial injury by immunologic factors rather than direct virally mediated endothelial injury. Direct damage to endothelial cells caused by viral-induced cytolysis is not described as the cause of bleeding diathesis in Ebola virus infection [29]. Multisystem organ failure affecting the hematopoietic, neurologic, and pulmonary systems often accompanies the vascular involvement. Hepatic involvement varies with the infecting organism and is at times seen with Ebola, Marburg, as well as other VHF agents, such as yellow fever. Renal failure with oliguria, although a prominent feature of hemorrhagic fever with renal syndrome (HFRS) seen in Hantavirus infection [30], may be seen in other VHF infections as intravascular volume depletion becomes more pronounced. Bleeding complications are particularly prominent with Ebola, Marburg, and the South American arenaviruses.

Clinical presentation

Although data exist from laboratory-based VHF infection in animal models, most clinical information regarding VHF infection comes from naturally occurring outbreaks. Suspicion for VHF infection in areas where these viruses are endemic should be high for patients who present even with nonspecific symptoms of viral infection, such as high fever, headache, fatigue, myalgias, abdominal pain, and non-bloody diarrhea. This constellation of symptoms has been well described during the initial prodromal period of VHF infection [3]. Following the terrorist incidents in September 2001, the CDC released instructions for recognizing illness associated with the release of a biologic agent, and listed clinical findings associated with Marburg and Ebola virus infection such as abrupt onset of fever, headache, and myalgias, followed by nausea, vomiting, abdominal pain, chest pain, and macular-papular rash, particularly involving the trunk [31]. Although this clinical presentation may not raise the specter of VHF infection in a routine emergency department setting in the United States or Europe, several recent cases of imported VHF infection from endemic areas to industrialized countries have been reported [32–34]. The ease and rapidity of global travel has likely increased the spread of unusual pathogens, including VHF agents.

In August 2004, a businessman who had made several recent trips to Liberia and Sierra Leone in West Africa presented to a New Jersey emergency department with fever of 103.6°F (39.8°C), chills, sore throat, diarrhea, and back pain. His condition deteriorated rapidly during hospitalization, requiring intubation, and mechanical ventilation. Diagnoses considered included yellow fever and Lassa fever, as well as typhoid fever and malaria. Despite aggressive supportive therapy, the patient died. Postmortem examination confirmed the diagnosis of Lassa fever by serum antigen detection, viral culture, and reverse transcriptase polymerase chain reaction (RT-PCR) assay. None of the patient's identified contacts either within the hospital or before his hospitalization reported symptoms consistent with Lassa virus infection [34].

The incubation period for VHF agents ranges from 2 to 21 days. The nonspecific prodromal symptoms of VHF infection noted above are often variable and differ between VHF agents as well. Filoviruses, such as Ebola and Marburg, tend to have a more rapid onset of symptoms; arenavirus infection may have a slower progression [3]. Because the target of VHF infection is the vascular system, symptoms of endothelial damage and increased vascular permeability tend to predominate. In early infection, patients present with conjunctival injection, mild hypotension, flushing, and petechial rash; in later stages of the disease, frank mucous membrane hemorrhage with shock and generalized bleeding may occur. Involvement of neurologic, pulmonary, and hematopoietic systems may also occur [35]. In Lassa fever, hemorrhagic complications tend to be less common than in filovirus infection. Deafness is a common long-term complication of significant Lassa fever infection. Evidence of hepatic injury such as jaundice is seen in Ebola, Marburg, and yellow fever.

Morbidity and mortality associated with VHF infection can be highly variable. During the 1995 Ebola (strain: Ebola-Zaire) outbreak in Kikwit, Democratic Republic of Congo, the case fatality rate was 81% [36]. During the 2000–2001 Uganda outbreak, the case fatality rate was just above 50%. The strain of Ebola isolated during the Uganda outbreak was Ebola-Sudan, one of four Ebola subtypes previously described. The others include the most virulent, Ebola-Zaire, with case fatality rates of 80%–90%, Ebola-Cote D'Ivoire, and Ebola-Reston (a variant first described in 1989 in Reston, Virginia, that only appears to affect nonhuman primates) [24].

Arenavirus infection typically results in mortality rates of 15%–20% for Lassa fever and 15%–30% for the New World arenaviruses [14,37]. Most patients (80%) with Lassa fever have either mild or no observable symptoms, and severe disease occurs in only 20% of those infected [38]. The mode of VHF exposure has been correlated with degree of illness. Particularly in filovirus infection, percutaneous acquisition of the disease is strongly correlated with increased mortality. During the 1976 Ebola-Zaire outbreak, every case of infection caused by contaminated syringes resulted in death [39].

In an African or South American health care setting, the diagnosis of VHF infection is far more likely than in an industrialized nation. Because of the infrequency of VHF illness in industrialized countries, the initial evaluation of a patient with suspected imported VHF infection should not only attempt to provide supportive therapy or specific antiviral agents as appropriate, but also to rule out other, more common, pathogens that may have specific therapies. The differential diagnosis of VHF encompasses a wide array of both infectious and non-infectious etiologies. Viral and bacterial illnesses that may mimic VHF include influenza, viral hepatitis, staphylococcal or gram-negative sepsis, meningococcemia, salmonellosis and shigellosis, as well as less common infections such as leptospirosis, malaria, rickettsial diseases (such as Rocky Mountain spotted fever), dengue, and hantavirus. Non-infectious causes that can cause bleeding diathesis include disseminated intravascular coagulation (DIC), idiopathic or thrombotic thrombocytopenic purpura, hemolytic-uremic syndrome, acute leukemia, and collagen-vascular diseases [3].

Potentially significant delays in the diagnosis of VHF infection are likely related to the rarity of these infections in the setting of routine emergency department or ICU care. In naturally occurring cases of VHF infection, patients generally have a history of travel to locales where VHF infection is endemic such as West or Central Africa, or South America, or have had contact with infected people or animals, or arthropod vectors, as in yellow fever. In the case of a bioterrorist attack, no warning would likely be forthcoming and the presentation of numbers of febrile patients with various nonspecific constitutional symptoms would be difficult to link to a common infectious source. During the 2001 anthrax bioterrorism attack, a shared route of exposure served to identify infected individuals as well as those who were potentially at risk for infection [40]. The virulence of these infectious agents and the special containment procedures required to handle them safely can introduce significant delays in definitive diagnosis. Hospital microbiology laboratories and local public health facilities are not equipped to diagnose VHF infection, and samples must be sent to either the Centers for Disease Control and Prevention (Atlanta, Georgia) or the US Army Medical Research Institute of Infectious Diseases (USAMRIID; Frederick, Maryland).

In the event of a bioterrorist attack involving large numbers of infected patients, a triage system would have to be enacted to allocate available health care resources to meet patient demand. Because of the rapid progression of disease, particularly in patients with filovirus infection, it has been difficult to establish which patients have the greatest chance for survival. Following an average incubation time of 5–7 days for Ebola or Marburg infection, the onset of disease is rapid; death usually occurs within 6–9 days of the onset of illness [41]. During the 2000–2001 Ebola outbreak in Uganda, a temporary diagnostic laboratory was established on-site, which was able to perform rapid, next-day, testing for Ebola virus by viral antigen capture ELISA and RT-PCR [42]. A retrospective analysis of the data obtained by this field laboratory also demonstrated that viral load correlated with disease outcome. Viral RNA copy levels in patients who died were 100 times higher than among those who survived the infection. RNA copy levels of 10^8/mL or higher were associated with a fatal outcome; the positive predictive value was >90%. Although somewhat intuitive (ie, patients who demonstrated evidence of overwhelming viremia did worse than those who did not), these data suggest some potential guidelines for the management of a mass casualty incident involving VHF infection. VHF patients (at least those with confirmed filovirus infection) with documented evidence of severe viremia are unlikely to benefit from the most aggressive resuscitative measures. Potentially saving these resources for those patients with a better chance of survival may result in improved overall survival among infected patients.

Designed for use in rural health care settings with limited resources, the set of guidelines for the care of VHF patients created jointly by the CDC and the World Health Organization can serve as a model for appropriate patient care that minimizes risk to health care providers and other non-infected persons and

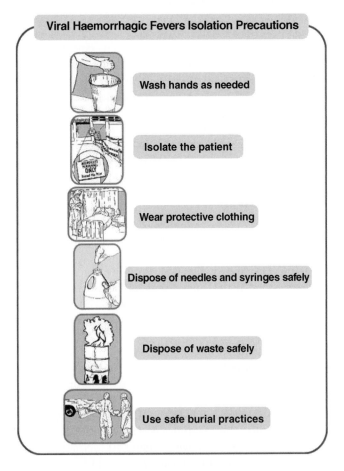

Fig. 1. Viral hemorrhagic fever isolation precautions. This basic set of isolation precautions for patients with suspected or confirmed VHF infection was developed by the CDC and the World Health Organization for instruction of health care providers in Africa. (*From* Centers for Disease Control and Prevention and World Health Organization. Infection control for viral haemorrhagic fevers in the African health care setting. Atlanta (GA): Centers for Disease Control and Prevention; 1998. Figs. 7, 26; with permission.)

optimizes use of available resources [43] (Fig. 1). In African filovirus outbreaks, infected patients have been grouped into isolation wards with separate areas for health care personnel to change into protective clothing. In industrialized countries, more resources are typically available and isolation precautions are generally required for only one or two patients. In the setting of a bioterrorism attack involving a VHF agent, however, significant numbers of symptomatic patients may be expected. Because of the potential severity of illness, estimation of the numbers of patients requiring critical care is difficult. Case fatality rates for VHF agents vary from 15% to as high as 90%, which suggests that the number of infected patients who might require critical care services is likely to represent at least 50% of symptomatic patients and perhaps nearly all patients with the most virulent forms of filovirus infection.

The need for intensive care for these patients has been clearly demonstrated in recently described cases of imported VHF [34,44]. In 2000, a nurse who was hospitalized with VHF symptoms (and was later diagnosed with Ebola-Zaire) in South Africa developed severe hemorrhagic complications and ultimately died of intracerebral hemorrhage. Before her death, she required prolonged intensive care (including 12 days of mechanical ventilation) as well as significant fluid resuscitation and blood product infusions. She underwent multiple invasive procedures, including two laparotomies, hemodialysis, pulmonary artery catheterization, and vasopressor infusion for persistent hypotension. This patient was cared for at Johannesburg Hospital, in an intensive care unit specifically designated for patients with hemorrhagic fevers. Careful attention to strict barrier precautions was likely responsible for the absence of any further transmission of the illness during the patient's hospitalization [44,45].

Decontamination and isolation

An essential priority for health care facilities and personnel caring for patients with confirmed or suspected VHF infection is containment of the disease. Both the filoviruses and arenaviruses are highly infectious through direct contact with blood and bodily secretions. Given the risk to health care providers demonstrated during previous naturally occurring VHF outbreaks, institution of appropriate barrier precautions and negative pressure isolation for these patients is vital. During the 1995 Ebola outbreak in Kikwit, Democratic Republic of Congo, 90 (32%) of 283 infected patients whose occupations were known, were identified as health care workers [46]. The initiation of barrier-nursing precautions during this outbreak was highly effective: only one health care worker became ill after the institution of preventive measures [37] (Fig. 2).

Any suspected case of VHF fever should be reported to the hospital epidemiologist or infection control officer as well as to local and state public health officials. Laboratory directors and personnel should also be notified so that additional precautions can be instituted amongst laboratory personnel. Notification of the CDC is essential in any case of suspected VHF infection to expedite

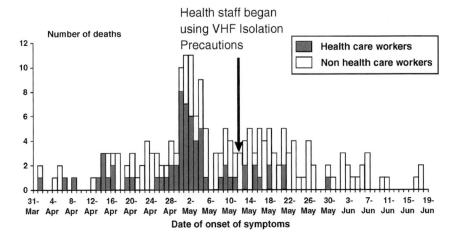

Fig. 2. The number of infected health care workers declined after barrier nursing practices were begun during the Ebola hemorrhagic fever outbreak at Kikwit, Democratic Republic of Congo, 1995. (*From* Centers for Disease Control and Prevention and World Health Organization. Infection control for viral haemorrhagic fevers in the African health care setting. Atlanta (GA): Centers for Disease Control and Prevention; 1998. Figs. 1, 3; with permission.)

virus-specific diagnostic testing and mobilize appropriate resources for containment and epidemiology [1]. Identification of specific VHF agents is beyond the scope of hospital laboratories and poses substantial risks to laboratory personnel because of the highly infectious nature of these viruses. Even in specialized facilities equipped to handle these agents, accidents have occurred resulting in unintended infection and death [47,48].

Specific infection-control recommendations for care of patients with suspected or confirmed VHF infection include: (1) Strict adherence to hand washing, (2) double gloving and the use of impermeable gowns, (3) N-95 masks or powered air-purifying respirators, (4) negative pressure isolation with 6–12 air exchanges per hour, (5) leg and shoe coverings, and (6) face shields or goggles. Additional containment measures include restricted access by nonessential staff and visitors, dedicated medical equipment for each patient such as stethoscopes, blood pressure cuffs, and if available, point-of-care analyzers, and environmental disinfection with hospital disinfectant approved by the Environmental Protection Agency or 1:100 bleach solution. Multiple potentially infected patients should be placed in the same part of the hospital to minimize exposure to other patients and health care workers. In the event of a mass casualty incident, even large nonpatient-care spaces can be converted into negative pressure areas through the use of portable high-efficiency particulate air filtered forced-air equipment [49]. Multiple studies of infection control measures instituted during VHF outbreaks have documented the efficacy of strict barrier-control measures in markedly reducing or eliminating the risk of disease transmission [14,21,23,32,50–52].

Patients who have survived VHF infection may remain contagious for extended periods of time during convalescence. Semen samples of Ebola survivors have demonstrated evidence of Ebola virus by RT-PCR 90 days after disease onset, although no live virus could be isolated [53]. Patients who have died of VHF infection should be promptly cremated or buried. Any unnecessary contact with the corpse including autopsy or embalming should be avoided. All contacts of patients diagnosed with VHF infection, including hospital personnel and laboratory workers, should be placed under medical surveillance for signs of VHF infection for 21 days (the theoretical maximal incubation period for VHF infection) [1,34].

Diagnostic studies

Hospital laboratories at major academic medical centers lack the capability to safely handle VHF agents. Patient samples must be specially handed and packaged for shippment to authorized laboratories for analysis. Only USAMRIID and CDC currently have the Biosafety Level-4 (BSL-4) laboratory resources to make virus-specific diagnoses of VHF infection [1]. The increased demand for BSL-4 containment facilities for bioterrorism research has recently led to a planned expansion of BLS-3 and BSL-4 facilities, including two new BSL-4-rated National Biocontainment Laboratories at Boston University and the University of Texas Medical Branch in Galveston, both funded by the National Institutes of Health [54].

Because of the barriers inherent in virus-specific testing, a case definition of presumptive VHF infection has been developed in the setting of naturally occurring VHF outbreaks using specific clinical diagnostic criteria (Box 1). The case definition developed for Ebola virus infection after the 1995 Kikwit outbreak uses the presence of fever and visible signs of bleeding, such as bleeding from gums, nose, conjunctival hemorrhage, ecchymosis, hematochezia, melena or hematemesis [43]. Other criteria include fever, with or without signs of bleeding, for persons who have contact with a patient with suspected Ebola virus infection. A clear, concise case definition for suspected VHF infection can serve as an appropriate initial screening tool in the setting of suspected VHF outbreak such as might be caused by an act of bioterrorism. In such a scenario, the large volume of patient specimens requiring definitive viral identification would likely be labor intensive and time consuming, potentially resulting in significant delays in diagnosis.

In specialized laboratories, virus-specific diagnoses of VHF agents can be made using several methods, including viral antigen-capture ELISA, RT-PCR, and viral isolation [3]. During the 1995 Kikwit Ebola outbreak, CDC researchers used viral antigen-capture ELISA assays as well as immunohistochemical staining of formalin-fixed tissue samples using a specific polyclonal antibody [46]. In recent filovirus outbreaks, field laboratories capable of performing viral antigen-capture ELISA as well as RT-PCR have been established to allow health care personnel access to highly specific diagnostic assays without substantial delays in specimen processing [42]. The use of a largely automated portable thermal cycler to prepare biological samples for DNA or RNA RT-PCR identification

Box 1. Case Definition, Ebola Hemorrhagic Fever (EHF)

Anyone presenting with fever and signs of bleeding such as:

- Bleeding of the gums
- Bleeding from the nose
- Red eyes
- Bleeding into the skin (purple colored patches in the skin)
- Bloody or dark stools
- Vomiting blood
- Other unexplained signs of bleeding

Whether or not there is a history of contact with a suspected case of EHF.
OR
Anyone living or deceased with:

- Contact with a suspected case of EHF AND
- A history of fever, with or without signs of bleeding.

OR
Anyone living or deceased with a history of fever AND 3 of the following symptoms:

- Headache
- Vomiting
- Loss of appetite
- Diarrhea
- Weakness or severe fatigue
- Abdominal pain
- Generalized muscle or joint pain
- Difficulty swallowing
- Difficulty breathing
- Hiccups

OR
Any unexplained death in an area with suspected cases of EHF.

(*From* Centers for Disease Control and Prevention and World Health Organization. Infection control for viral haemorrhagic fevers in the African health care setting. Atlanta (GA): Centers for Disease Control and Prevention; 1998. p. 145; with permission.)

has reduced potentially hazardous exposure by laboratory personnel to highly infectious biological agents [55,56].

For the diagnosis of Lassa fever, ELISA assays have recently proved as reliable as indirect fluorescent antibody testing, the previous standard method of viral identification [57]. Junin virus, the cause of Argentine hemorrhagic fever, has been identified using ELISA assays to detect Junin IgG antibodies in infected rodents [58]. More recently, PCR assays have become available for both Lassa and Junin, and a PCR has been developed that predictably amplifies any member of the Arenaviridae family by targeting a highly conserved RNA terminal segment [59].

Treatment

Treatment for VHF infection is primarily supportive. There are no antiviral drugs approved by the US Food and Drug Administration for use in the setting of VHF infection [3]; however, small published trials have shown that intravenous ribavirin, a nucleoside analog that markedly reduces levels of guanosine monophosphate, guanosine diphosphate, and guanosine triphosphate, has been used to treat Lassa fever with significant reduction in mortality [60]. Similar results have been shown using intravenous ribavirin for the treatment of some New World arenaviruses as well [61]. Ribavirin is available for compassionate use under an investigational new drug protocol.

No antiviral agents have proven effective against either Ebola or Marburg infection and development of a filovirus virus vaccine has been a significant focus of ongoing research efforts [62–65]. An Ebola DNA plasmid vaccine that relies on a DNA "primer" from three strains of Ebola virus recently completed NIH-sponsored Phase I human trials, and is in an active follow-up phase, however, no data are yet available [66,67]. Another team of researchers is currently focusing on an Ebola vaccine based on non-virulent Ebola virus proteins that stimulate both antibody- and T cell-mediated host immune responses [68]. This group has also described similar protection from Marburg virus infection using Marburg virus-like particles [69]. The Ebola protein-based vaccine is currently undergoing primate studies. The efficacy of an Ebola vaccine in humans will be understandably difficult to assess clinically given the unlikely scenario that healthy human volunteers would consent to being exposed to live wild-type Ebola virus, even if vaccinated [70].

Research into vaccines against Lassa virus and other New World arenaviruses are ongoing at CDC [71]. Although additional funding has recently become available for Lassa virus research, difficulty in conducting vaccine trials in endemic areas and lack of political stability in these regions remain significant obstacles to vaccine development and testing. A live attenuated virus vaccine against Argentine hemorrhagic fever (Junin) is available and effective, and may protect against Bolivian hemorrhagic fever (caused by Machupo virus) as well [34,72].

In the setting of a bioterrorist attack using a VHF bioweapon, vaccination is not a viable solution. Following vaccination, antibody titers tend to rise slowly, typically requiring months to confer full immunity. Treatment of persons already infected with VHF agents has been the subject of intense research interest, particularly given the increasing number of recent, naturally occurring filovirus outbreaks. The use of convalescent serum (ie, sera from patients who have survived infection) has been suggested as a possible therapy. Late during the 1995 Kikwit outbreak, eight Ebola patients received whole blood transfusions from Ebola survivors. Of these, seven survived. However, there is no clear evidence that links their survival directly to this therapy, and no clear demonstration of benefit can be generalized from these data [73]. The use of immune plasma has proved effective in the treatment of some arenaviruses, including Junin and Machupo, although difficulties with plasma collection and storage may limit the effectiveness of this therapy [74,75].

Novel antiviral regimens have had some success in in vitro studies against Lassa, Ebola and the Severe Acute Respiratory Syndrome (SARS) coronavirus [76]. In addition to blocking viral replication, recent efforts have attempted to target the VHF disease process itself by inhibiting the action of proinflammatory cytokines thereby attenuating the consumptive coagulopathy that is the hallmark of the disease [77]. Currently, however, there is no effective therapy for VHF infection other than ribavirin for patients with Lassa fever or New World arenavirus infection; treatment for filovirus infection remains supportive.

Supportive care

Treatment of the VHF-infected patient presents substantial difficulties, which are complicated by the need to maintain strict barrier controls to prevent the transmission of VHF infection to treating health care and laboratory personnel,. The need to administer fluids, electrolytes, and blood products is likely to be significant in these patients. In patients with Lassa fever, dehydration, edema, hypotension, and renal insufficiency are common [38]. The use of invasive procedures, however, should be minimized to reduce the risk to staff of iatrogenic transmission of a potentially lethal pathogen. In published descriptions of imported cases of VHF infection, the time to diagnosis is often significantly delayed. After returning from Sierra Leone in West Africa, a surgeon was hospitalized in the Netherlands with a working diagnosis of typhoid fever, and was not diagnosed with Lassa fever until day 13 and died 3 days later despite the initiation of ribavirin therapy [23]. After diagnosis, 128 unprotected contacts were identified; of the 83 investigated contacts, none showed seroconversion by Lassa virus antibody screen. Although the diagnosis in this case was delayed, methicillin-resistant *Staphylococcus aureus* (MRSA) contact isolation precautions had been instituted early during the patient's hospitalization.

The need for volume resuscitation in patients with VHF infection is greatest in late stages of infection, as patients develop worsening hemorrhage and shock.

It has been shown that viral loads also tend to be higher in later stages of infection, which may increase infectivity of blood or body fluids [42]. Despite the intuitive concept that the sickest patients may benefit the most from the highest level of care, there is no clear evidence that more vigorous resuscitation of severely symptomatic VHF patients leads to a decrease in mortality. During the Kikwit Ebola outbreak, however, an increased incidence of coughing and hemoptysis among survivors was thought perhaps to reflect increased use of parenteral fluid resuscitation later during the outbreak [78]. The data available regarding the care of VHF patients in modern emergency department and intensive care unit settings are confined to a few isolated case reports from which no clear generalization regarding improvement in patient outcomes can be derived. In recent naturally-occurring outbreaks of Ebola or Marburg virus, most of the patients were cared for in isolation wards, grouped together with similarly infected patients because of lack of individualized isolation, decontamination, and treatment facilities.

Clinical course and prognostic factors

A typical clinical course for patients with VHF infection cannot be generalized for all VHF patients as the causative organism is closely linked to the patient's clinical course and overall outcome. Some VHF agents, such as the arenaviruses, have a relatively low incidence of hemorrhagic side effects; others, such as Ebola and Marburg, tend to follow a more fulminant course. As previously noted, most patients with Lassa fever tend to have a mild clinical course, and those infected with Ebola-Zaire may experience a case fatality rate of 80%–90% [38,46].

The presence of significant volume depletion, coupled with hemodynamic instability is a poor prognostic sign in patients with VHF infection. In the largest case study of Ebola-Zaire infection, terminally ill patients typically presented with signs of severe volume loss, including obtundation, anuria, and shock [78]. Another finding noted in this case series was the premorbid finding of tachypnea. Among this group of patients, tachypnea was the most significant criteria differentiating between fatal and nonfatal outcomes ($P = 0.0027$) [78]. Tachypnea was generally associated with bleeding from mucosa and puncture sites, anuria and hiccups; the tachypnea preceded death by only a few days.

Prognostic factors associated with worse patient outcomes have also been derived from field-based genetic studies of VHF agents, as well as the presence or absence of certain clinical signs or symptoms. RT-PCR assays and quantitative analysis of RNA viral load in patients infected with Ebola-Sudan during the 2000–2001 Uganda outbreak were used retrospectively to identify those patients more likely to have a fatal outcome [42]. The presence of edema (typically accompanied by dehydration and hypotension) has been identified as a poor prognostic sign in patients with Lassa fever [38]. A review of pediatric Lassa fever cases identified a "swollen baby syndrome" consisting of widespread edema, abdominal distension, and bleeding that ended in death in three of four cases. Its absence is thought to be a good prognostic factor in children with Lassa fever [79].

Unfortunately, the largest clinical studies of VHF patients have been derived from an imperfect combination of highly sensitive laboratory-based viral assays, and unreliable or incomplete clinical data obtained during naturally occurring outbreaks in rural Third World health care settings. These complex interdependent factors complicate the development of rigorous, evidence-based conclusions regarding the expected clinical course or prognostic factors for VHF patients in an urban, industrialized hospital setting where state-of-the-art emergency department and intensive care resources are readily available.

Summary

The previously unthinkable prospect of bioterrorism has become, in the post September 11 political climate, a proven threat that presents a substantial, ongoing risk to industrialized nations. This risk requires a healthy respect for the capabilities of the most lethal potential agents of bioterrorism, in this case, the viral hemorrhagic fevers. These lethal viruses represent a continuing public health threat in endemic areas. Now, because of the ease and speed of global travel, business travelers and tourists unwittingly infected with these deadly pathogens are arriving without warning at hospitals in industrialized nations, presenting novel diagnostic challenges—as well as significant new risks— to western health care workers and hospital employees. By recognizing risk factors for both naturally acquired VHF infection as well as signs and symptoms of a VHF-based bioterrorism attack, physicians and other health care workers who use proper barrier precautions can evaluate and manage patients suspected of harboring VHF infection and at the same time minimize the infectious risk of these highly contagious and potentially lethal pathogens.

References

[1] Centers for Disease Control and Prevention. Update: management of patients with suspected viral hemorrhagic fever—United States. MMWR Morb Mortal Wkly Rep 1995;44(25):475–9.
[2] Centers for Disease Control and Prevention. Biological and chemical terrorism: strategic plan for preparedness and response. Recommendations of the CDC Strategic Planning Workgroup. MMWR Recomm Rep 2000 Apr 21;49(RR-4):1–14.
[3] Borio L, Inglesby T, Peters CJ, et al. Hemorrhagic fever viruses as biological weapons: medical and public health management. JAMA 2002;287(18):2391–405.
[4] Davis CJ. Nuclear blindness: An overview of the biological weapons programs of the former Soviet Union and Iraq. Emerg Infect Dis 1999;5(4):509–12.
[5] Alibek K, Handelman S. Biohazard: the chilling true story of the largest covert biological weapons program in the world, told from the inside by the man who ran it. New York: Random House; 1999.
[6] Okumura T, Suzuki K, Fukuda A, et al. The Tokyo subway sarin attack: disaster management, Part 1: community emergency response. Acad Emerg Med 1998;5(6):613–7.

[7] Global Proliferation of Weapons of Mass Destruction. Hearings Before the Permanent Subcommittee on Investigations of the Committee on Governmental Affairs, United States Senate, 104th Cong, 1st–2nd Sess (1996).

[8] Jaax N, Jahrling P, Geisbert T, et al. Transmission of Ebola virus (Zaire strain) to uninfected control monkeys in a biocontainment laboratory. Lancet 1995;346(8991–8992):1669–71.

[9] Johnson E, Jaax N, White J, et al. Lethal experimental infections of rhesus monkeys by aerosolized Ebola virus. Int J Exp Pathol 1995;76(4):227–36.

[10] Leffel EK, Reed DS. Marburg and Ebola viruses as aerosol threats. Biosecur Bioterror 2004; 2(3):186–91.

[11] Centers for Disease Control and Prevention. Outbreak of Ebola hemorrhagic fever Uganda, August 2000-January 2001. MMWR Morb Mortal Wkly Rep 2001;50(5):73–7.

[12] Stephenson EH, Larson EW, Dominik JW. Effect of environmental factors on aerosol-induced Lassa virus infection. J Med Virol 1984;14(4):295–303.

[13] Carey DE, Kemp GE, White HA, et al. Lassa fever. Epidemiological aspects of the 1970 epidemic, Jos, Nigeria. Trans R Soc Trop Med Hyg 1972;66(3):402–8.

[14] Charrel RN, de Lamballerie X. Arenaviruses other than Lassa virus. Antiviral Res 2003; 57(1–2):89–100.

[15] Lehmann-Grube F. Portraits of viruses: arenaviruses. Intervirology 1984;22(3):121–45.

[16] Banerjee K, Gupta NP, Goverdhan MK. Viral infections in laboratory personnel. Indian J Med Res 1979;69:363–73.

[17] Rouquet P, Froment J-M, Bermejo M, et al. Wild animal mortality monitoring and human Ebola outbreaks, Gabon and Republic of Congo, 2001–2003. Emerg Infect Dis 2005;11(2): 283–90.

[18] Centers for Disease Control and Prevention. Update: filovirus infection associated with contact with nonhuman primates or their tissues. MMWR Morb Mortal Wkly Rep 1990;39(24):404–5.

[19] Peterson AT, Carroll DS, Mills JN, et al. Potential mammalian filovirus reservoirs. Emerg Infect Dis 2004;10(12):2073–81.

[20] Zaki SR, Shieh WJ, Greer PW, et al. A novel immunohistochemical assay for the detection of Ebola virus in skin: implications for diagnosis, spread, and surveillance of Ebola hemorrhagic fever. Commission de Lutte contre les Epidemies a Kikwit. J Infect Dis 1999;179(Suppl 1): S36–47.

[21] Colebunders R, Sleurs H, Pirard P, et al. Organisation of health care during an outbreak of Marburg haemorrhagic fever in the Democratic Republic of Congo, 1999. J Infect 2004; 48(4):347–53.

[22] International Society for Infectious Diseases. Hemorrhagic fever— Angola: Marburg virus confirmed, March 22, 2005 [Archive no. 20050322.0831]. Available at: http://www.promedmail. org. Accessed March 10, 2005.

[23] Swaan CM, van den Broek PJ, Kampert E, et al. Management of a patient with Lassa fever to prevent transmission. J Hosp Infect 2003;55(3):234–5.

[24] Peters CJ, LeDuc JW. An introduction to Ebola: the virus and the disease. J Infect Dis 1999;179(Suppl 1):ix–xvi.

[25] Peters CJ, Zaki SR. Role of the endothelium in viral hemorrhagic fevers. Crit Care Med 2002;30(5 Suppl):S268–73.

[26] Villinger F, Rollin PE, Brar SS, et al. Markedly elevated levels of interferon (IFN)-gamma, IFN-alpha, interleukin (IL)-2, IL-10, and tumor necrosis factor-alpha associated with fatal Ebola virus infection. J Infect Dis 1999;179(Suppl 1):S188–91.

[27] Feldmann H, Bugany H, Mahner F, et al. Filovirus-induced endothelial leakage triggered by infected monocytes/macrophages. J Virol 1996;70(4):2208–14.

[28] Geisbert TW, Hensley LE, Larsen T, et al. Pathogenesis of Ebola hemorrhagic fever in cynomolgus macaques: evidence that dendritic cells are early and sustained targets of infection. Am J Pathol 2003;163(6):2347–70.

[29] Geisbert TW, Young HA, Jahrling PB, et al. Pathogenesis of Ebola hemorrhagic fever in primate models: evidence that hemorrhage is not a direct effect of virus-induced cytolysis of endothelial cells. Am J Pathol 2003;163(6):2371–82.

[30] Lee HW. Hemorrhagic fever with renal syndrome in Korea. Rev Infect Dis 1989;11 (May–Jun):S864–76.

[31] Centers for Disease Control and Prevention. Recognition of illness associated with the intentional release of a biologic agent. MMWR Morb Mortal Wkly Rep 2001;50(41):893–7.

[32] Haas WH, Breuer T, Pfaff G, et al. Imported Lassa fever in Germany: surveillance and management of contact persons. Clin Infect Dis 2003;36(10):1254–8.

[33] Hugonnet S, Sax H, Pittet D. Management of viral haemorrhagic fevers in Switzerland. Euro Surveill 2002;7(3):42–4.

[34] Centers for Disease Control and Prevention (CDC). Imported Lassa fever–New Jersey, 2004. MMWR Morb Mortal Wkly Rep 2004;53(38):894–7.

[35] Jahrling P. Viral hemorrhagic fevers. In: Zajtchuk R, Bellamy RF, editors. Textbook of military medicine: medical aspects of chemical and biological warfare. Chapter 29. Washington DC: Office of the Surgeon General; 1989. p. 591–602.

[36] Khan AS, Tshioko FK, Heymann DL, et al. The reemergence of Ebola hemorrhagic fever, Democratic Republic of the Congo, 1995. Commission de Lutte contre les Epidemies a Kikwit. J Infect Dis 1999;179(Suppl 1):S76–86.

[37] McCormick JB, King IJ, Webb PA, et al. A case-control study of the clinical diagnosis and course of Lassa fever. J Infect Dis 1987;155(3):445–55.

[38] Richmond JK, Baglole DJ. Lassa fever: epidemiology, clinical features, and social consequences. BMJ 2003;327(7426):1271–5.

[39] World Health Organization. Ebola haemorrhagic fever in Zaire, 1976. Bull World Health Organ 1978;56(2):271–93.

[40] Centers for Disease Control and Prevention. Update: investigation of bioterrorism-related anthrax and adverse events from antimicrobial prophylaxis. MMWR Morb Mortal Wkly Rep 2001;50(44):973–6.

[41] Bray M. Defense against filoviruses used as biological weapons. Antiviral Res 2003;57(1–2): 53–60.

[42] Towner JS, Rollin PE, Bausch DG, et al. Rapid diagnosis of Ebola hemorrhagic fever by reverse transcription-PCR in an outbreak setting and assessment of patient viral load as a predictor of outcome. J Virol 2004;78(8):4330–41.

[43] Centers for Disease Control and Prevention, World Health Organization. Infection control for viral haemorrhagic fevers in the African health care setting. Atlanta (GA): Centers for Disease Control and Prevention; 1998. p. 1–198.

[44] Richards GA, Murphy S, Jobson R, et al. Unexpected Ebola virus in a tertiary setting: clinical and epidemiologic aspects. Crit Care Med 2000;28(1):240–4.

[45] Gradon J. An outbreak of Ebola virus: lessons for everyday activities in the intensive care unit. Crit Care Med 2000;28(1):284–5.

[46] Centers for Disease Control and Prevention. Update: outbreak of Ebola viral hemorrhagic fever–Zaire, 1995. MMWR Morb Mortal Wkly Rep 1995;44(25):468–9, 475.

[47] Barry M, Russi M, Armstrong L, et al. Brief report: treatment of a laboratory-acquired Sabia virus infection. N Engl J Med 1995;333(5):294–6.

[48] International Society for Infectious Diseases. Ebola, lab accident death - Russia (Siberia), May 22, 2004. [Archive no. 20040522.1377]. Available at: http://www.promedmail.org. Accessed March 10, 2005.

[49] Rosenbaum RA, Benyo JS, O'Connor RE, et al. Use of a portable forced air system to convert existing hospital space into a mass casualty isolation area. Ann Emerg Med 2004;44(6):628–34.

[50] Crowcroft NS, Meltzer M, Evans M, et al. The public health response to a case of Lassa fever in London in 2000. J Infect 2004;48(3):221–8.

[51] Communicable Disease Surveillance Centre. Lassa fever imported to England. Commun Dis Rep CDR Wkly 2000;10(11):99.

[52] Lamunu M, Lutwama JJ, Kamugisha J, et al. Containing a haemorrhagic fever epidemic: the Ebola experience in Uganda (October 2000-January 2001). Int J Infect Dis 2004;8(1):27–37.

[53] Rowe AK, Bertolli J, Khan AS, et al. Clinical, virologic, and immunologic follow-up of convalescent Ebola hemorrhagic fever patients and their household contacts, Kikwit, Demo-

cratic Republic of the Congo. Commission de Lutte contre les Epidemies a Kikwit. J Infect Dis 1999;179(Suppl 1):S28–35.

[54] NIAID funds construction of biosafety laboratories. Available at http://www.nih.gov/news/pr/sep2003/niaid-30.htm. Accessed March 10, 2005.

[55] Weidmann M, Muhlberger E, Hufert FT. Rapid detection protocol for filoviruses. J Clin Virol 2004;30(1):94–9.

[56] Drosten C, Kummerer BM, Schmitz H, et al. Molecular diagnostics of viral hemorrhagic fevers. Antiviral Res 2003;57(1–2):61–87.

[57] Bausch DG, Rollin PE, Demby AH, et al. Diagnosis and clinical virology of Lassa fever as evaluated by enzyme-linked immunosorbent assay, indirect fluorescent-antibody test, and virus isolation. J Clin Microbiol 2000;38(7):2670–7.

[58] Morales MA, Calderon GE, Riera LM, et al. Evaluation of an enzyme-linked immunosorbent assay for detection of antibodies to Junin virus in rodents. J Virol Methods 2002;103(1):57–66.

[59] Gunther S, Emmerich P, Laue T, et al. Imported lassa fever in Germany: molecular characterization of a new lassa virus strain. Emerg Infect Dis 2000;6(5):466–76.

[60] McCormick JB, King IJ, Webb PA, et al. Lassa fever. Effective therapy with ribavirin. N Engl J Med 1986;314(1):20–6.

[61] Enria DA, Maiztegui JI. Antiviral treatment of Argentine hemorrhagic fever. Antiviral Res 1994;23(1):23–31.

[62] Geisbert TW, Hensley LE. Ebola virus: new insights into disease aetiopathology and possible therapeutic interventions. Expert Rev Mol Med 2004;6(20):1–24.

[63] Geisbert TW, Jahrling PB. Towards a vaccine against Ebola virus. Expert Rev Vaccines 2003; 2(6):777–89.

[64] Sullivan NJ, Sanchez A, Rollin PE, et al. Development of a preventive vaccine for Ebola virus infection in primates. Nature 2000;408(6812):605–9.

[65] Hart MK. Vaccine research efforts for filoviruses. Int J Parasitol 2003;33(5–6):583–95.

[66] Vastag B. Ebola vaccines tested in humans, monkeys. JAMA 2004;291(5):549–50.

[67] NIAID Ebola vaccine enters human trial. Available at http://www.niaid.nih.gov/newsroom/releases/ebolahumantrial.htm. Accessed March 10, 2005.

[68] Warfield KL, Bosio CM, Welcher BC, et al. Ebola virus-like particles protect from lethal Ebola virus infection. Proc Natl Acad Sci USA 2003;100(26):15889–94.

[69] Warfield KL, Swenson DL, Negley DL, et al. Marburg virus-like particles protect guinea pigs from lethal Marburg virus infection. Vaccine 2004;22(25–26):3495–502.

[70] Gibbs WW. An uncertain defense. How do you test that a human Ebola vaccine works? You don't. Sci Am 2004;291(4):20, 24.

[71] Fisher-Hoch SP, McCormick JB. Lassa fever vaccine. Expert Rev Vaccines 2004;3(2):189–97.

[72] Maiztegui JI, McKee Jr KT, Barrera Oro JG, et al. Protective efficacy of a live attenuated vaccine against Argentine hemorrhagic fever. J Infect Dis 1998;177(2):277–83.

[73] Mupapa K, Massamba M, Kibadi K, et al. Treatment of Ebola hemorrhagic fever with blood transfusions from convalescent patients. J Infect Dis 1999;179(Suppl 1):S18–23.

[74] Enria DA, Briggiler AM, Fernandez NJ, et al. Importance of dose of neutralising antibodies in treatment of Argentine haemorrhagic fever with immune plasma. Lancet 1984;2(8397):255–6.

[75] Harrison LH, Halsey NA, McKee Jr KT, et al. Clinical case definitions for Argentine hemorrhagic fever. Clin Infect Dis 1999;28(5):1091–4.

[76] Gunther S, Asper M, Roser C, et al. Application of real-time PCR for testing antiviral compounds against Lassa virus, SARS coronavirus and Ebola virus in vitro. Antiviral Res 2004; 63(3):209–15.

[77] Geisbert TW, Hensley LE, Jahrling PB, et al. Treatment of Ebola virus infection with a recombinant inhibitor of factor VIIa/tissue factor: a study in rhesus monkeys. Lancet 2003; 362(9400):1953–8.

[78] Bwaka MA, Bonnet MJ, Calain P, et al. Ebola hemorrhagic fever in Kikwit, Democratic Republic of the Congo: clinical observations in 103 patients. J Infect Dis 1999;179(Suppl 1):S1–7.

[79] Monson MH, Cole AK, Frame JD, et al. Pediatric Lassa fever: a review of 33 Liberian cases. Am J Trop Med Hyg 1987;36(2):408–15.

ELSEVIER
SAUNDERS

CRITICAL
CARE
CLINICS

Crit Care Clin 21 (2005) 785–813

Radiation

John W. Burnham, PhD*, Janet Franco, MS

*Environmental Health and Radiation Safety, Oregon Health and Science University,
3181 SW Sam Jackson Park Road, Portland, OR 97239-3098, USA*

The US Department of Energy Radiation Emergency Assistance Center/ Training Site (REAC/TS) accident registry indicates that from 1944 to December 2004, there have been 427 radiation accidents involving significant radiation exposure to 3050 individuals [1]. This number includes United States and non-United States accidents. However, radiation is rarely used as a weapon. Chechen rebels reportedly placed a container of radioactive cesium in a Moscow park, to demonstrate their capability to news media, although there were no documented radiation injuries [2]. In 2003, the *Washington Times* reported that a suspected Al Qaida terrorist was being sought by the Federal Bureau of Investigation and the Central Intelligence Agency in connection with the acquisition of Canadian nuclear material to construct a "dirty bomb" [3].

These events, and other recent acts of domestic terrorism involving chemical and biological agents, have led to heightened concern about whether America is prepared to respond to a large-scale event. Radiation as a weapon of terrorism focuses on the use of nuclear weapons, improvised nuclear devices, or radio-logical dispersal devices (RDD). Some authors also propose the possible covert use of a gamma source placed in a busy public place, referred to as a "simple radiological device," or the release of radioactivity from a direct attack on a nuclear power plant [4]. However, an RDD is the most likely weapon of terror, because of its relatively simple technology and the widespread use of radioactive materials at industrial and research facilities and hospitals [5].

RDD is the term often used to refer to a dirty bomb, although several other means of disseminating radioactive material exist, many of which do not require explosives. The term dirty bomb generally refers to the combination of ra-

---

* Corresponding author.
E-mail address: burnhamj@ohsu.edu (J.W. Burnham).

0749-0704/05/$ – see front matter © 2005 Elsevier Inc. All rights reserved.
doi:10.1016/j.ccc.2005.06.003   *criticalcare.theclinics.com*

dioactive isotopes and high explosives which combine to spread radioactivity over a large area. This term was first used publicly in June 2002, by the United States Attorney General during an announcement of the arrest of Jose Padilla, who was charged with the construction of such a device.

An RDD has yet to be used as a weapon of terror and so it is not clear what the impact of such a weapon would be. The tragic event in Goiania, Brazil, may serve as the closest model for a stealth RDD attack as no overt event occurred [6,7]. Likewise, the Chernobyl nuclear power plant incident may be a good model for the worst-case scenario of an attack on a nuclear power plant. Still, there is disagreement about the likely outcome of a large radiological event. Some experts believe it would be very difficult, using an RDD with conventional explosives, to disperse radioactive material sufficient to produce high dose rates and result in serious injury [6]. Hence, attacks involving an RDD or a simple radiological device used surreptitiously may have the potential to cause more radiation injuries, whereas a dirty bomb RDD may elicit more immediate public fear and panic.

The incident in Goiania, Brazil, had widespread impact. Scrap metal scavengers unknowingly released an estimated 50.9 TBq of ^{137}Cs (cesium-137) from a stored medical source. Over several days, the glowing blue powder found its way into numerous homes and buildings. A total of 249 people were confirmed to be directly effected by radiation; of these, 151 exhibited internal contamination, including 46 who were treated with Prussian blue. Ultimately, 28 individuals suffered radiation burns and 4 people died of infectious and hemorrhagic complications. One of the fatalities was a 6-year-old girl who played with the powder and consumed a contaminated sandwich. Six homes were demolished, and 42 had to be evacuated for decontamination. Decontamination was required for shops, bars, and pavement in 58 public places, along with 64 vehicles. In the process, 3500 m^3 of radioactive waste was collected. Negative economic consequences ensued for the region and interregional trade declined.

Mechanism of toxicity

In the event of an accident, it is likely that the source of exposure and contamination will be known; however, at the time of an act of terrorism, and for several hours afterwards, the source may be unidentified. This can delay accurate estimates of absorbed doses and knowledge of the physiologic system(s) at greatest risk.

As a result of an explosion involving radioactive materials, or from radioactive particles downwind of a release, victims may become exposed to external radiation without becoming contaminated, or they may become externally contaminated by direct contact with radioactive material. In the case of airborne or loose radioactivity, the contamination may be inhaled, ingested, or incorporated through open wounds, which results in internal contamination.

Radiation interactions in tissue occur randomly. Initially, all damage occurs at the molecular level with variable impact. Manifest damage is seen when the physiologic function of large numbers of cells for a given tissue or organ are sufficiently altered [8].

Most initial interactions occur with water molecules, which make up 70%–80% of the cell. These interactions can result in ionization of water molecules producing a free electron and a positively charged water molecule, or a hydrogen ion and a hydroxyl radical. Through a series of steps, other free radicals may be created. Some of these entities may directly cause organelle or cellular damage through oxidative processes and can result in the formation of hydrogen peroxide.

Ionization by particles such as fast (high-energy) neutrons and high-energy alpha particles occurs when these particles interact in tissue, slow rapidly and deposit their energy over relatively short paths. These high linear-energy-transfer (LET) particles also possess high relative biological effectiveness (RBE) and inflict more shallow biologic damage than penetrating radiation such as gamma rays. RBE compares a dose of the standard energy of x-rays required to produce a given effect, with a dose of some other radiation type and energy.

Radiation can also ionize atoms within macromolecules, such as proteins and DNA. This may break covalent bonds, changing the biologic or chemical function of the macromolecule. This damage is not necessarily fatal to the cell and may be repaired. DNA is one of the most sensitive molecular targets and, if damage is not repaired correctly, the result can be genetic effects in later generations or cell death. This damage is in the form of single- and double-strand breaks [9]. With single-strand breaks, the intact complementary strand is available as a template to copy the damaged section. Although repair of double-strand breaks does occur, only a fraction will be without error.

Although alpha particles have high LET and high RBE, they do not penetrate deeply, and result in very shallow tissue damage. Alpha particles do not penetrate clothing and travel only fractions of a millimeter in tissue; consequently, they are normally only of concern in cases of internal contamination. Gamma rays, x-rays, and neutrons, largely because of their lack of charge, penetrate much deeper. Tissue penetration by beta particles is dependent on beta particle energy.

Absorbed dose is the deposition of energy in matter per unit mass. The international unit for absorbed dose is the gray (Gy). A related unit, which accounts for the ability of the radiation to damage tissue, is the sievert (Sv) or equivalent dose. For gamma rays and beta particles, these are numerically equivalent. Sv is commonly used when referring to internal contamination.

Predicting the outcome of a radiation exposure is complicated because of the many variables that must be estimated. Exposure to ionizing radiation can have short- and long-term human health effects, and are cumulative [5]. The deterministic effects of radiation are dependent on radiation type, total dose, whether the dose received was acute or chronic, distance from the source, protective clothing or barrier present at the time of exposure, portion of body exposed, and medical care. Potential deterministic effects include local radiation injury, acute radiation syndrome, and in utero abnormalities. One stochastic effect is cancer, although radiation induced carcinomas are indistinguishable from those caused by other agents.

Clinical presentation

Acute radiation syndrome (ARS) is caused by whole body exposure (WBE), or exposure of a significant portion of the body, to a high dose of penetrating radiation over a short period of time. Several studies are available that identify the classical symptoms and symptom sequence associated with ARS, or the synonymous term acute radiation sickness [10–14]. Current studies are largely based on past reports describing radiation accidents and detonation of atomic weapons. ARS pathogenesis stems from damage to predecessor cell fractions of various radiosensitive tissues. These include hematopoietic cells, cells lining the intestinal crypts and vascular endothelium. Consequently, the clinical components of ARS can include hematopoietic, gastrointestinal, and neurovascular syndromes. Each of these syndromes may be divided into four phases. Hence, some authors present ARS symptoms in the context of prodromal, latent, manifest illness, and recovery or death phases [10,11]. Dose and dose rate directly influence the severity and timing of symptoms in each stage. The potential for involvement of multiple physiologic systems dictates that ARS should be viewed as the interplay of all exhibited pathologies.

A cutaneous syndrome often occurs in conjunction with ARS, and can potentially alter the course of ARS progression [11]. Diagnosis and prognosis are complicated by the likelihood of uneven distribution of dose, differences in relative biological effectiveness for different radiations, and tissue specific sensitivity to radiation. Prognosis improves substantially in instances of relatively uniform exposure combined with laboratory findings.

Acute radiation syndrome

The prodromal phase (Table 1) after WBE often lasts only 24–48 hours and is normally characterized by the relatively rapid onset of vomiting, nausea, and malaise, with diarrhea at higher levels of exposure [12]. Temporary or permanent sterility may also be present [5]. The clinical picture most often resembles that of an acute viral illness, which makes diagnosis difficult in the absence of confirmed radiation exposure. This phase of ARS also exhibits the initiation of the hematopoietic syndrome at exposures ≥ 0.5–1.0 Gy [10,13].

Following the prodromal phase, a relatively asymptomatic latent phase (Table 2) of up to 5 or 6 weeks ensues. The duration of this phase is directly related to total dose and may last less than 1 day or be nonexistent at very high exposure levels. The large variability in the duration of the latent phase makes it impractical to hospitalize all patients suspected of radiation injury during the latency period. Further development of immunosuppression also characterizes this phase at moderate and higher exposures; the reduction in absolute lym-

Table 1
Prodromal phase of acute radiation syndrome

Symptoms and medical response	ARS degree and the approximate dose of acute WBE (Gy)				
	Mild (1–2)	Moderate (2–4)	Severe (4–6)	Very severe (6–8)	Lethal[a] (>8)
Vomiting					
Onset	2 h after exposure or later	1–2 h after exposure	Earlier than 1 h after exposure	Earlier than 30 min after exposure	Earlier than 10 min after exposure
% of incidence	10–50	70–90	100	100	100
Diarrhea	None	None	Mild	Heavy	Heavy
Onset	—	—	3–8 h	1–3 h	Within minutes or 1 h
% of incidence	—	—	<10	>10	Almost 100
Headache	Slight	Mild	Moderate	Severe	Severe
Onset	—	—	4–24 h	3–4 h	1–2 h
% of incidence	—	—	50	80	80–90
Consciousness	Unaffected	Unaffected	Unaffected	May be altered	Unconsciousness (may last sec/min)
Onset	—	—	—	—	Sec/min
% of incidence	—	—	—	—	100 (at >50 Gy)
Body temperature	Normal	Increased	Fever	High fever	High fever
Onset	—	1–3 h	1–2 h	<1 h	<1 h
% of incidence	—	10–80	80–100	100	100
Medical response	Outpatient observation	Observation in general hospital, treatment in specialized hospital if needed	Treatment in specialized hospital	Treatment in specialized hospital	Treatment in specialized hospital[b]

[a] With appropriate supportive therapy individuals may survive whole body doses of approximately 10 Gy.

[b] For absorbed dose above 10 Gy, palliative treatment is appropriate.

Adapted from International Atomic Energy Agency. Diagnosis and treatment of radiation injuries. Safety Reports Series No. 2. Vienna: IAEA; 1998.

Table 2
Latent phase of acute radiation syndrome

	Degree of ARS and approximate dose of acute WBE (Gy)				
	Mild (1–2)	Moderate (2–4)	Severe (4–6)	Very severe (6–8)	Lethal (>8)
Lymphocytes (G/L) (days 3–6)	0.8–1.5	0.5–0.8	0.3–0.5	0.1–0.3	0.0–0.1
Granulocytes (G/L)	>2.0	1.5–2.0	1.0–1.5	≤0.5	≤0.1
Diarrhea	None	None	Rare	Appears on days 6–9	Appears on days 4–5
Epilation	None	Moderate, beginning on day 15 or later	Moderate or complete on days 11–21	Complete earlier than day 11	Complete earlier than day 10
Latency period (d)	21–35	18–28	8–18	7 or less	None
Medical response	Hospitalization not necessary	Hospitalization recommended	Hospitalization necessary	Hospitalization urgently necessary	Hospitalization urgently necessary[a]

[a] For absorbed dose above 10 Gy, palliative treatment is appropriate.
Adapted from International Atomic Energy Agency. Diagnosis and treatment of radiation injuries. Safety Reports Series No. 2. Vienna: IAEA; 1998.

Table 3
Manifest illness phase of acute radiation syndrome

	Degree of ARS and approximate dose of acute WBE (Gy)				
	Mild (1–2)	Moderate (2–4)	Severe (4–6)	Very severe (6–8)	Lethal (>8)
Onset of symptoms (d)	>30	18–28	8–18	<7	<3
Lymphocytes (G/L)	0.8–1.5	0.5–0.8	0.3–0.5	0.1–0.3	0.0–0.1
Platelets (G/L) (%)	60–100	30–60	25–35	15–25	<20
	10–25	25–40	40–80	60–80	80–100[a]
Clinical manifestations	Fatigue, weakness	Fever, infections, bleeding, weakness, epilation	High fever, infections, bleeding, epilation	High fever, diarrhea, vomiting, dizziness and disorientation, hypotension	High fever, diarrhea, unconsciousness
Lethality (%)	0	0–50	20–70	50–100	100
		Onset 6–8 weeks	Onset 4–8 weeks	Onset 1–2 weeks	Onset 1–2 weeks
Medical response	Prophylactic	Special prophylactic treatment from days 14–20; isolation from days 10–20	Special prophylactic treatment from days 7–10; isolation from the beginning	Special treatment from day 1; isolation from the beginning	Special treatment from day 1; isolation from the beginning[b]

[a] In very severe cases, with a dose of >50 Gy, death precedes cytopenia.
[b] For absorbed dose above 10 Gy, palliative treatment is appropriate.

Adapted from International Atomic Energy Agency. Diagnosis and treatment of radiation injuries. Safety Reports Series No. 2. Vienna: IAEA; 1998.

phocyte count presents a very useful measure of radiation exposure intensity. Latency transitions into acute and manifest illness.

Table 3 presents the severity of symptoms in the manifest illness stage. Lethal dose in 50% of patients 60 days post exposure ($LD_{50/60}$) may be observed during this stage at moderate doses in the absence of supportive therapy [13,15]. Moderate and higher doses often present thrombocytopenia induced bleeding diathesis. At these higher levels of exposure, injury to the gastrointestinal tract may begin to overlap the bone marrow syndrome, and the gastrointestinal syndrome may become the dominant feature at much higher doses (10–15 Gy) [10]. Yet higher doses yield an irreversible neurovascular syndrome.

Patients who survive this critical period make clear progress toward recovery in most cases, typically over a period of months, and gradually return to normal hematological parameters. Occasionally, recovery may take up to 2 years [11]. Survivors must also face the potential for stochastic effects. Appropriate medical care will likely result in an $LD_{50/60}$ between 6–7 Gy; the maximum survivable dose is about 10 Gy [13,15]. Lymphocyte decline after high dose exposure occurs predictably. A potential lethal injury is indicated by a 50% reduction in absolute lymphocytes in the first 24 hours, followed by a second more severe drop within 48 hours. The basis of a lethal outcome is normally irreversible hematopoiesis damage leading to sepsis, hemorrhage, pneumonia, and multiple organ failure.

An alternative presentation of ARS symptoms was recently discussed in a consensus review by the Strategic National Stockpile Radiation Working Group available at www.bt.cdc.gov/radiation/ [13]. Outcomes are presented based on the degree of severity of hematologic change for the hematopoietic system (Table 4) and for the gastrointestinal, neurovascular, and cutaneous systems (Table 5). The signs and symptoms related to the severity of injury to each of these systems are valuable for patient triage, therapy, and assignment of prognosis. The same authors also approximated the time course for expression of hematopoietic, gastrointestinal, and neurovascular symptoms at different WBE dose ranges (Fig. 1).

Cutaneous syndrome

Several studies indicate that accidental radiation exposures leading to localized injury are often associated with WBE and occur more frequently [10,16–20]. Many of these localized injuries involve the hand (Fig. 2) and can be sufficiently serious to complicate the course and management of ARS (Fig. 3). There are prominent differences between the cutaneous syndrome (CS; sometimes called local radiation injury or cutaneous radiation syndrome) and ARS: the substantially higher absorbed dose required to induce significant CS, and the prolonged time for onset of symptoms (Table 6). One clinical characteristic always associated with CS is injury to the stem cells of the skin, which leads to dry or moist desquamation at sufficiently high doses. Skin injuries resemble thermal burns; however, the volume of tissue involved with CS can be much larger because of underlying tissue damage. This phenomena leads to a delay in the

Table 4
Levels of hematopoietic toxicity

Symptom or sign	Degree 1	Degree 2	Degree 3	Degree 4
Lymphocyte changes[a]	$\geq 1.5 \times 10^9$ cells/L	$1-1.5 \times 10^9$ cells/L	$0.5-1 \times 10^9$ cells/L	$<0.5 \times 10^9$ cells/L
Granulocyte changes[b]	$\geq 2 \times 10^9$ cells/L	$1-2 \times 10^9$ cells/L	$0.5-1 \times 10^9$ cells/L	$<0.5 \times 10^9$ cells/L
Thrombocyte changes[c]	$\geq 100 \times 10^9$ cells/L	$50-100 \times 10^9$ cells/L	$20-50 \times 10^9$ cells/L	$<20 \times 10^9$ cells/L
Blood loss	Petechiae, easy bruising, normal hemoglobin level	Mild blood loss with $<10\%$ decrease in hemoglobin level	Gross blood loss with 10%–20% decrease in hemoglobin level	Spontaneous bleeding or blood loss with $>20\%$ decrease in hemoglobin level

[a] Reference value, $1.4-3.5 \times 10^9$ cells/L.
[b] Reference value, $4-9 \times 10^9$ cells/L.
[c] Reference value, $140-400 \times 10^9$ cells/L.

Adapted from Fliedner TM, et al. Medical management of radiation accidents: manual on the acute radiation syndrome. Oxford: British Institute of Radiology; 2001; with permission. Also see reference [13].

Table 5
Grading system for response of neurovascular, gastrointestinal, and cutaneous systems

Symptom	Degree 1	Degree 2	Degree 3	Degree 4
Gastrointestinal system				
Diarrhea				
Frequency (stools/d)	2–3	4–6	7–9	≥ 10
Consistency	Bulky	Loose	Loose	Watery
Bleeding	Occult	Intermittent	Persistent	Persistent with large amount
Abdominal cramps or pain	Minimal	Moderate	Intense	Excruciating
Neurovascular system				
Nausea	Mild	Moderate	Intense	Excruciating
Vomiting	Occasional (once per d)	Intermittent (2–5 times/d)	Persistent (6–10 times/d)	Refractory (> 10 times/d)
Anorexia	Able to eat	Intake decreased	Intake minimal	Parenteral nutrition
Fatigue syndrome	Able to work	Impaired work ability	Needs assistance from ADLs	Cannot perform ADLs
Temperature (°C)	<38	38–40	>40 for <24 h	>40 for <24 h
Headache	Minimal	Moderate	Intense	Excruciating
Hypotension	Heart rate > 100 beats/min; blood pressure > 100/170 mm Hg	Blood pressure <100/170 mm Hg	Blood pressure <90/60 mm Hg; transient	Blood pressure <80/? mm Hg; persistent

Neurologic deficits[a]	Barely detectable	Easily detectable	Prominent	Life-threatening, loss of consciousness
Cognitive deficits[b]	Minor loss	Moderate loss	Major impairment	Complete impairment
Cutaneous system				
Erythema[c]	Minimal, transient	Moderate (<10% body surface area)	Marked (10%–40% body surface area)	Severe (>40% body surface area)
Sensation or itching	Pruritus	Slight and intermittent pain	Moderate and persistent pain	Severe and persistent pain
Swelling or edema	Present, asymptomatic	Symptomatic, tension	Secondary dysfunction	Total dysfunction
Blistering	Rare, sterile fluid	Rare, hemorrhage	Bullae, sterile fluid	Bullae, hemorrhage
Desquamation	Absent	Patchy dry	Patchy moist	Confluent moist
Ulcer or necrosis	Epidermal only	Dermal	Subcutaneous	Muscle or bone involvement
Hair loss	Thinning, not striking	Patchy, visible	Complete, reversible	Complete, irreversible
Onycholysis	Absent	Partial	Partial	Complete

Abbreviation: ADL, activity of daily living.

[a] Reflex status (including corneal reflexes), papilledema, seizures, ataxia, and other motor signs or sensory signs.

[b] Impaired memory, reasoning, or judgment.

[c] The extent of involvement is decisive and should be documented for all skin changes.

Adapted from Fliedner TM, et al. Medical management of radiation accidents: manual on the acute radiation syndrome. Oxford: British Institute of Radiology; 2001; with permission. See also reference [13].

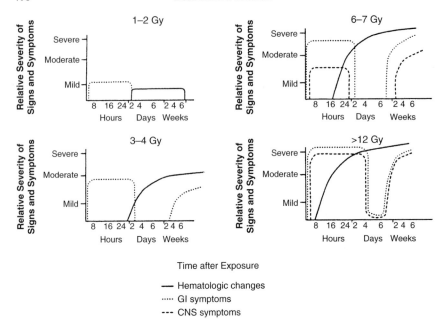

Time after Exposure

— Hematologic changes
····· GI symptoms
- - - CNS symptoms

Fig. 1. Approximate time course of clinical manifestations. Shown are approximate times for hematopoietic, gastrointestinal (GI), and central nervous system symptoms at different ranges of dose of whole-body radiation for exposed, living persons. Hematopoietic changes include development of lymphopenia, granulocytopenia, or thrombocytopenia. GI symptoms include headache, nausea, vomiting, or diarrhea. Cerebrovascular signs and symptoms include headache, impaired cognition, disorientation, ataxia, seizures, prostration, and hypotension. Note that the signs and symptoms of different organ systems significantly overlap at each radiation dose and that cerebrovascular symptoms do not appear until exposure to a high whole-body dose. The relative severity of signs and symptoms is measured on an arbitrary scale. (*Adapted from* Waselenko JK, MacVittie TJ, Blakely WF, et al. Medical management of acute radiation syndrome: recommendations of the strategic national stockpile radiation looking group. Ann Intern Med 2004;140(12):1037–51; with permission.)

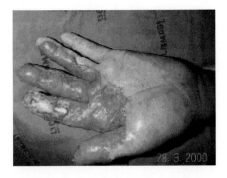

Fig. 2. Severe local radiation injury eight weeks after handling 15.7 TBq of ^{60}Co. (*Adapted from* International Atomic Energy Agency. The radiological accident in Samut Prabarn. Vienna: IAEA; 2002; with permission.)

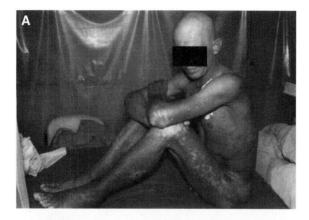

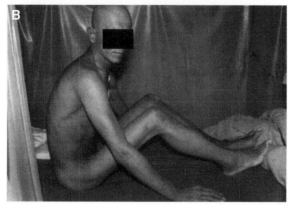

Fig. 3. Cutaneous syndrome with acute radiation syndrome 74 days after 11 Gy dose to ^{60}Co source: (*A*) left side; (*B*) right side. (*Adapted from* International Atomic Energy Agency. The radiological accident at the irradiation facility in Nesvizh. Vienna: IAEA; 1996; with permission.)

onset of clinical changes (Table 6) and can result in substantial impairment [10,12,13].

CS is heavily influenced by the degree of penetration of ionizing radiation. Generally, only gamma, neutron, and higher energy beta radiation exhibit significant penetration. Severity of injury has been classified in grades I–IV [18] and separately, correlated with dose [10,12]. For continuity of discussion, symptoms related to estimated dose and the associated phases are discussed.

Comparatively low dose exposures (6–8 Gy) can result in prodromal symptoms of warmth, itching, or mild erythema, followed by a latent phase of several weeks. The skin becomes reddened in the manifest illness phase and dry desquamation may occur, progressing to complete recovery.

Higher doses (8–15 Gy) are characterized by acute CS syndrome wherein the prodromal stage includes itching, pain, erythema, and dry desquamation. The latent phase generally lasts 1–2 weeks, followed by what appears to be a second-

Table 6
Time of onset of clinical signs of skin injury depending on the dose received

Stage/symptoms	Dose range (Gy)	Time of onset (d)
Erythema	3–10	14–21
Epilation	>3	14–18
Dry desquamation	8–12	25–30
Moist desquamation	15–20	20–28
Blister formation	15–25	15–25
Ulceration (within skin)	>20	14–21
Necrosis (deeper penetration)	>25	>21

Adapted from International Atomic Energy Agency. Diagnosis and treatment of radiation injuries. Safety Reports Series No. 2. Vienna: IAEA; 1998.

degree thermal burn. These injuries are quite painful, susceptible to infection, and slow to heal.

Much higher doses (>20 Gy) present rapidly appearing erythema with associated intense pain in a very short prodromal phase, quickly yielding blisters with resultant wet desquamation and ulceration. Depth of injury resembles a thermal third-degree burn, which likely requires grafting. Involvement of an extremity may require amputation. Injury of the cutaneous system is always present in CS; however, penetrating doses in this range can also lead to dilatation and alteration of blood capillaries, as well as damage to arterial vessels, cartilage, bone, muscles, and nerves [18].

In circumstances of non-uniform exposure leading to both ARS and CS, the course of ARS can be substantially altered [11]. Gamma exposures >30 Gy over more than 25% of the body, or 50 Gy to 10%–15% of the body surface, result in critical medical status. This is further enhanced if high dose regions include the head, chest, or abdomen.

Differential diagnosis

Early diagnosis of either CS or ARS will likely present a challenge for the clinician, especially in the absence of knowledge of possible radiation exposure. CS must be considered in the differential diagnosis if the patient presents with a skin lesion and no history of thermal or chemical burn, insect bite, allergy, or skin disease. Smith and colleagues [21] indicate that CS skin lesions have been mistaken for pemphigus.

Knowledge of possible radiation exposure, or finding and handling an unknown metallic object, combined with erythema, blistering, dry or wet desquamation, epilation, or ulceration can be indicative of CS. Also, as mentioned earlier, CS skin injuries are slow to evolve and heal. Conventional wound management may be ineffective and consultation with radiation experts is recommended [22].

The signs and symptoms of ARS are non-specific and easily confused with those of other illnesses or injuries. Strong similarities exist with acute viral infection, gastroenteritis, and pancytopenia [10,12,21]. ARS should be considered in the differential diagnosis when there is a history of possible radiation exposure, lymphopenia, neutropenia, and thrombocytopenia (especially when combined with respiratory infection), a tendency to bleed (epistaxis, petechiae), or epilation. Any of these combined with unexplained nausea and vomiting during the previous few weeks is indicative. Ultimate diagnosis may require clinical assay of dicentrics in peripheral blood lymphocytes. The reality of successful differential diagnosis of CS and ARS, is that the clinician may need to have a "stronger index of suspicion" [21].

Radiologic terrorism impact

Numerous views of the potential outcomes of a terrorist act involving radioisotopes have been presented. The Centers for Disease Control [21] recently itemized five possible scenarios for radiation terrorism:

- Nuclear weapon
- Improvised nuclear device
- Nuclear power-plant incident
- Hidden source of radiation (simple radiological device)
- Dirty bomb

A nuclear weapon or improvised nuclear device requires the most sophistication and cost to produce and generates the greatest hazard [23]. Nuclear detonation results in the most devastation, casualties, and long-term effects, compared with other radiologic weapons. The blast moves away from the point of detonation at roughly the speed of sound, and the thermal effects will travel at the speed of light. The distance at which an immediate radiation dose—in the mid-lethal range—is delivered, increases with the power of the bomb. The blast site will remain radioactive for years because of the presence of long half-life radioisotopes and the radioactive particles (fallout) that will be dispersed over large distances. Environmental conditions impact the number of non-blast related illnesses.

The unlikely event of a successful attack or sabotage on a nuclear reactor, resulting in cooling system failure, could also have catastrophic results. The results of a massive reactor event are evident from the Chernobyl disaster and the subsequent release of huge quantities of highly radioactive, airborne particles.

Simple radiologic devices containing high-energy, long-lived ^{137}Cs or ^{60}Co (cobalt-60) could easily be placed in a busy pedestrian area [4]. There have been numerous reports of stolen industrial gauges that contain these radioactive sources. Radiologic dispersal devices (RDD), constructed using isotopes common in hospitals, could use ^{137}Cs, ^{60}Co, ^{131}I (radioactive iodine), or ^{90}Sr (strontium) [24]. However, it is estimated that the source used must contain substantial activity (at least 3.7 TBq) before radiation injuries are likely to result.

The diversity of opinions concerning the impact of a terrorist act involving one of these scenarios no doubt stems from the following variables:

- Varying assessments of the security of facilities and sources
- Level of technical expertise required for device assembly
- Quantity and specific isotope used
- Form of the isotope (powder, pellets, liquid, and so forth)
- Facilities required for device assembly
- Health risk during assembly of a workable device
- Potential for detection
- Environmental factors (wind and so on) influencing outcome

These barriers, along with the obvious fiscal barrier, present a substantial, tangible challenge to an individual or group intent on pursuing an act of radiologic terrorism. Subjectively, one can conclude that short of assistance from a willing country or entity with adequate knowledge and resources, or the improbable event of a successful attack on a nuclear power plant [25], it is unlikely that a radiologic incident resulting in large numbers of radiation-induced casualties will occur. Following this logic, the most likely scenarios would be those using the simplest technology.

It is beyond the scope of this article to systematically explore the likelihood and potential outcomes of all possible scenarios. However, estimates of the number of casualties resulting from some of the potential scenarios have been made [26–29]. The Department of Homeland Security has projected that the scope of patients that could require evaluation or treatment after the use of an RDD would be <1000. For an improvised nuclear device, the estimate is >100,000. No doubt, many of those requiring evaluation would be "worried well." Fatality estimates for these two scenarios are tens to hundreds and tens of thousands respectively; essentially all RDD fatalities are related to an initial explosion. The Strategic National Stockpile Radiation Working Group estimates a 1-kiloton nuclear detonation in a city of 2 million would result in >7000 fatalities, 1000–3000 combined injuries, 136,500 radiation fallout exposures requiring medical care, and >150,000 people who require monitoring for psychological well-being [13].

The Health Physics Society and a recent report to Congress agree that immediate health effects from an RDD event, other than from an associated explosion, would be minimal [27,28]. The use of a simple radiological device is likely to expose only a handful of victims [21]. More recently, the Homeland Security Council (HSC) estimated that an RDD using explosives could result in 180 fatalities, 270 injuries, 20,000 individuals with detectable superficial contamination, and 50,000 worried well [29]. They also concluded that "no one will suffer ARS." HSC estimates that casualties would vary widely for an improvised nuclear device.

Considering the range of current estimates, if the subjective conclusion that a terrorist act is likely to use the simplest technology is accurate, then it could be further projected that patients needing evaluation would be a minimum of 1000, and a much smaller number (possibly nil) would need treatment for CS or ARS. This conclusion should be evaluated and balanced with the fact that the Goiania, Brazil, incident resulted in 112,000 persons being monitored and 249 who were contaminated internally or externally. The inescapable conclusion is that in the absence of an act of nuclear terrorism, the number of individuals requiring some level of critical care would likely be a few hundred or less, although the number of worried well requiring evaluation could easily be several thousand. In addition, the number of critical care patients suffering some degree of radiation injury could be very limited and dependent upon the specific radionuclide and its activity, the means of dissemination, or the geographical location of a hidden source.

Radiation injury medical management

Medical management of radiation casualties includes proper preparation for receipt of victims, triage, and emergency care. Psychosocial assistance will likely be required for any significant radiological event. During initial assessment and triage, victims are identified as having external or internal contamination, significant external exposure with no contamination, or injuries caused by trauma. Consultation with a hematologist, burn specialist, dermatologist, neurologist, or trauma surgeon may also be required for comprehensive assessment. Definitive assessment should lead to treatment and supportive care for patients exhibiting ARS, internal contamination, and combined radiation injury.

Hospital preparations

Emergency departments must take immediate steps once notified of incoming potential radiation victims [4,12,21,30]. The reader is referred to other articles [12,30] for in-depth coverage of emergency room (ER) management involving radiation injured patients. Essential steps include:

- Assemble treatment team
- Notify hospital administration and local authorities
- Review radiological incident procedures/equipment/kits
- Assume patients are contaminated
- Arrange radiation monitoring assistance
- Establish preplanned treatment area near outside entrance
- Determine "background" radiation of treatment area
- Remove or cover equipment that will not be needed
- Provide large plastic-lined containers for contaminated material and clothing
- Cover treatment table with several layers of waterproof, disposal sheeting
- Assume full universal precautions by emergency room personnel

- Cover floor areas, leading to treatment area with taped absorbent pads or butcher paper, or transport contaminated patients wrapped in clean sheets
- Establish control line on clean side of entrance to treatment area
- Monitor to confirm contamination does not move to clean areas
- Provide dosimeters to all staff

Medical advice for the assessment and treatment of radiation casualties is available within the United States from REAC/TS (www.orau.gov/reacts/; 865-576-1005) and the Medical Radiobiology Advisory Team (301-295-0316).

Triage and emergency care

Triage is the practice of sorting individuals on the basis of their injury or illness in an effort to rapidly identify the level of medical care required for the largest number of people. In all likelihood, on-scene triage, radiological contamination assessment, and decontamination will occur for most victims before arrival at the medical facility. Upon arrival at the hospital, symptoms related to radiation exposure can initially serve as the basis of categorizing and treating

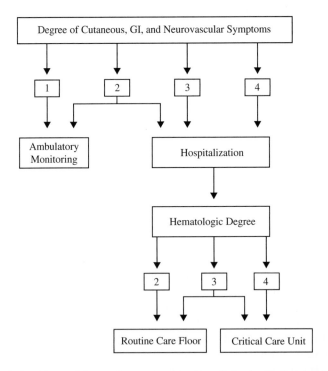

Fig. 4. Approach to triage and therapy for persons exposed to radiation in a limited-casualty scenario. (*Adapted from* Dainiak N. Hematologic consequences of exposure to ionizing radiation. Exp Hematol 2002;30:513–28; with permission.)

victims; however, prompt emergency treatment of life-threatening injuries always takes precedence.

The number of casualties may determine the triage process used. One approach to triage and treatment for a limited-casualty radiologic scenario uses an assessment of the level of injury (see Table 5) to the gastrointestinal, neurovascular, and cutaneous systems [13,31]. This assessment, combined with early estimates of the degree of toxicity to the hematopoietic system (see Table 4), provides a triage system (Fig. 4) for the selection of level of care. Further triage using biological dosimetry can greatly aid the clinician with definitive diagnosis. This approach is limited by laboratory turnaround time and may only be useful for a small number of victims.

A triage process can also be based on prodromal early clinical signs and symptoms such as vomiting, diarrhea, and erythema [10]. This approach can assist with the decision to hospitalize for both WBE and local exposure (LE), and can be effective when evaluating large numbers of casualties (Table 7). In addition, these signs and symptoms could be combined with other ARS prodromal observations, local exposure locations, thermal and trauma injuries, for use with a more sophisticated radiation casualty management software tool. Referred to as the Biological Assessment Tool, this software program was developed by the Armed Forces Radiobiology Research Institute (Bethesda, Maryland) and is available on their website at www.afrri.usuhs.mil/. Triage planning for a large-scale incident should also include preparations for expeditious assessment of the worried well, to provide timely critical care to victims with survivable injuries.

The triage system selected should always accommodate patients with combined injury. Categorization must include those individuals with significant trauma and burns. Surgical intervention required for combined injury should take place within the first 48 hours; subsequent surgery should be delayed 6–12 weeks [4,13]. Following is a list of priorities upon patient arrival at the ER in approximate order of importance:

- Administer lifesaving assistance
- Stabilize medical conditions
- Treat serious injuries before decontamination
- Collect any available information on patient radiation exposure
- Assess patient external contamination (Geiger-Muller survey meter)
- Document areas of contamination on body chart
- Decontaminate patient and treatment area
- Treat minor injuries
- Maintain treatment area containment
- Assess internal contamination
- Treat internal contamination
- Assess local radiation injuries

There is almost universal consensus that external patient contamination represents an extremely low risk to health care workers who observe universal

Table 7
Guide for the management of radiation injuries based on early symptoms

Clinical signs		Corresponding dose (Gy)		Decision
WBE	LE	WBE	LE	
No vomiting	No early erythema	<1	<10	Outpatient with 5 week surveillance period (blood, skin)
Vomiting 2–3 h after exposure	Early erythema or abnormal sensation 12–24 h after exposure	1–2	8–15	Surveillance in a general hospital (or outpatient for 3 weeks followed by hospitalization if necessary)
Vomiting 1–2 h after exposure	Early erythema or abnormal sensation 8–15 h after exposure	2–4	15–30	Hospitalization in a hematological or surgical (burn) department
Vomiting earlier than 1 h after exposure and/or other severe symptoms (eg, hypotension)	Early erythema, within the first 3–6 h (or less) after exposure, skin and/or mucosa with edema	>4	>30	Hospitalization in a well-equipped hematological or surgical department with transfer to a specialized center for radiopathology

Adapted from International Atomic Energy Agency. Diagnosis and treatment of radiation injuries. Safety Reports Series No. 2. Vienna: IAEA; 1998.

precautions [32]. It is difficult, if not impossible, for a patient to be so contaminated that they present a radiation hazard to health care workers who follow precautions [13,14]. The level of risk should be evaluated by the clinical radiation safety officer, radiologist, or nuclear medicine physician and communicated to medical caregivers. There is also general agreement that movement of contaminants from the treatment room into the hospital ventilation system is highly unlikely [33]. Staff stress may be alleviated through prior training on radiation basics and planned drills. Also effective are debriefing and counseling for staff and victims. Because one of the primary objectives of terrorism is to cause psychological shock, planning for the medical management of psychosocial symptoms is essential [13,14,32]. Individuals who are especially susceptible are pregnant women, children, mothers of young children, those with a prior history of psychiatric disorder, and family of exposed victims. Additional guidelines are available at: www.bt.cdc.gov/radiation/pdf/MassCasualtiesGuidelines.pdf.

Decontamination

One rule of thumb concerning patient decontamination is that removal of clothing is likely to eliminate up to 90% of external contamination [30]. Contaminated clothing should be placed in a clearly marked container (RADIOACTIVE – DO NOT DISCARD). Clothing removal combined with decontamination of skin surfaces and hair using warm water and mild soap generally removes 95% of contamination [14,26]. However, care should be taken when decontaminating thermal burns, to prevent the removal of marginally viable skin, which makes burn treatment more difficult. Contaminated areas should be resurveyed to determine if levels have been effectively reduced. Generally, levels equal to or greater than twice the background merit additional decontamination [12]. Wounds should be protected during skin decontamination and irrigated with sterile solution, which is removed via suction before performing any necessary debridement. Liquid wastes from decontamination should be contained only if practical [26]. Protective equipment should be carefully removed after use and placed in a labeled, sealed plastic container.

Internal contamination can result from ingestion, inhalation, or wounds involving radioactive material. Nasal swabs must be obtained as early as possible and counted, although nasal passage samples are subject to error from cross contamination. If contamination is present in both nostrils, inhalation should be assumed. Urine and feces samples are retained and monitored for contamination activity [26,34].

Diagnosis

Signs and symptoms, along with samples taken for laboratory evaluation (see Table 4) during triage, can help determine the initial management steps required.

Lab tests should include complete blood count (CBC) with differential count, routine chemistry, and a heparinized sample for cytogenetics [13,35].

Since the hematopoietic system exhibits the first indications of exposure severity, absolute lymphocyte, neutrophil, platelet, and erythrocyte counts are essential. Lymphocyte sensitivity is reflected by rapid, early decline and a nadir of 3–5 days post exposure. CBC repeated every 4–6 hours can be used to evaluate lymphocyte depletion kinetics. Neutrophil decrease is more gradual with nadir at 4–6 weeks. Platelets and red blood cells are relatively radioresistant with platelets requiring WBE of 2.0–5.0 Gy to reach counts leading to bleeding diathesis. Anemia is not commonly observed during ARS because of red blood cell life span.

Peripheral lymphocyte chromosomal studies should be conducted as early as 24 hours after exposure because of rapid lymphocyte decline. Cytogenetic analysis for chromosome aberrations (dicentrics) is time consuming and results may not be available for 48 to 72 hours after the sample is submitted.

The prodromal onset time of vomiting combined with blood data on lymphocyte depletion and frequency of lymphocyte dicentrics represent an effective means of biodosimetry. These three parameters have been combined (Table 8) to assist with absorbed dose estimates [13].

CS with or without ARS will result in cutaneous injury and may involve deeper structures. If physical dosimetry is not available, electron spin resonance (ESR) can be useful for estimating dose. ESR methods applied to solid materials such as teeth and clothing, measure free radicals formed by ionizing radiation [18]. Additional diagnostic procedures used to estimate severity of local exposures are thermography and radioisotope methods. Thermography measures the infrared radiation emitted from skin surfaces [36]. Distortions in the thermal symmetry of the normal body can be identified and the extent of the lesion defined. Vascular circulation can be recorded using technetium-99 metastable pertechnate injected intravenously, and then monitoring distribution via scintillation camera [37].

Assessment and diagnosis of internal contamination should be undertaken in the first few hours after exposure for maximum treatment effectiveness. Often, available facts are limited leading up to early decisions to treat for internal radioisotopes. One essential component is the determination of whether the incorporated isotope is a beta-gamma or an alpha emitter. This should be discernable using the appropriate Geiger-Muller survey instruments. Nasal swabs, and urine and feces samples, combined with the level of skin and clothing contamination, can give a rough idea of the amount of radioactivity present. The decision to initiate treatment very early post-exposure may require a best estimate of whether the exposure potential is low, medium, or high, although one author has proposed that treatment for equivalent doses below 0.1–0.5 Sv may be of limited value [34]. This combined with knowledge of the risk or reward associated with treatment, may allow treatment to be initiated while waiting for more detailed evaluation of dose. The reader is referred to work by Voelz [34] for detailed coverage of internal contamination.

Table 8
Biodosimetry based on acute photon-equivalent exposures

Dose estimate	Victims with vomiting	Time to onset of vomiting	Absolute lymphocyte count[a]						Rate constant for lymphocyte depletion[b]	Dicentrics in human peripheral blood lymphocytes[c]	
			Day 0.5	Day 1	Day 2	Day 4	Day 6	Day 8		Per 50 cells	Per 1000 cells
Gy	%	h	× 10⁹ cells/L						k§	n	
0	—	—	**2.45**	**2.45**	**2.45**	**2.45**	**2.45**	**2.45**	—	0.05–0.1	1–2
1	19	—	**2.30**	**2.16**	**1.90**	**1.48**	1.15	0.89	0.126	4	88
2	35	4.63	**2.16**	**1.90**	**1.48**	0.89	0.54	0.33	0.252	12	234
3	54	2.62	**2.03**	**1.68**	1.15	0.54	0.25	0.12	0.378	22	439
4	72	1.74	**1.90**	**1.48**	0.89	0.33	0.12	0.044	0.504	35	703
5	86	1.27	**1.79**	1.31	0.69	0.20	0.06	0.020	0.63	51	1024
6	94	0.99	**1.68**	1.15	0.54	0.12	0.03	0.006	0.756		
7	98	0.79	**1.58**	1.01	0.42	0.072	0.012	0.002	0.881		
8	99	0.66	**1.48**	0.89	0.33	0.044	0.006	<0.001	1.01		
9	100	0.56	1.39	0.79	0.25	0.030	0.003	<0.001	1.13		
10	100	0.48	1.31	0.70	0.20	0.020	0.001	<0.001	1.26		

Dose range is based on acute photon-equivalent exposures. The second column indicates the percentage of people who vomit, based on dose received and time to onset. The middle section depicts the time frame for development of lyphopenia. Blood lymphocyte counts are determined twice to predict a rate constant that is used to estimate exposure dose. The final column represents the current gold standard, which requires several days before results are known. Colony-stimulating factor therapy should be initiated when onset of vomiting or lymphocyte depletion kinetics suggests an exposure dose above 2 Gy. Therapy may be discontinued if results from chromosome dicentrics analysis indicate a lower estimate of whole-body dose.

[a] Normal range, 1.4–3.5 × 10⁹ cells/L. Numbers in boldface fall within this range.

[b] The lymphocyte depletion rate is based on the model $Lt = 2.45 \times 10^9$ cells/L $\times$ e − k(D)t, where Lt equals the lymphocyte count ($\times 10^9$ cells/L), 2.45×10^9 cells/L equals a constant representing the consensus mean lymphocyte count in the general population, k equals the lymphocyte depletion rate constant for a specific acute photon dose, and t equals the time after exposure (days).

[c] Number of dicentric chromosomes in human peripheral blood lymphocytes.

Adapted from Waselenko JK, MacVittie TJ, Blakely WF, et al. Medical management of the acute radiation syndrome: recommendations of the strategic national stockpile radiation working group. Ann Intern Med 2004;140(12):1037–51.

Acute radiation syndrome treatment

The high radiosensitivity of stem and progenitor cells of the hematopoietic system can result in lymphopenia and bone marrow atrophy. Although these manifestations are not clinically significant below 1 Gy, WBE >2–3 Gy can result in acute expression [38].

The relatively large size of the human body and proximity to the source can lead to non-uniform absorbed dose. At severe exposure levels, this phenomenon can play a major role in the reconstitution of hematopoiesis through minimal damage to some regions of bone marrow. Dose reconstruction may be difficult and combined injuries are likely to occur when events involve nuclear detonation, which complicates ARS management. Immunosuppression will in turn complicate wound and burn healing.

First and foremost in the treatment of ARS is careful observation of early signs and symptoms combined with lymphocyte depletion results over the first 48 hours. Lymphocyte depletion represents the single most useful data point to estimate injury severity. These observations, especially when combined with lymphocyte dicentrics, can provide dose estimates used for treatment guidance (Tables 8 and 9).

Cytokine therapy

Recommended cytokines include granulocyte-colony stimulating factor (G-CSF) and granulocyte macrophage-colony stimulating factor (GM-CSF) in conjunction with interleukin IL-3 [10]. More recently, pegylated G-CSF has also been recognized as a therapeutic option [13,38]. Although, these cytokines have not been approved for treatment of aplasia from radiation exposure, the rationale for using CSF is based on several observations. These include improved survival for irradiated experimental animals (including nonhuman primates), enhanced neutrophil recovery in cancer patients, and an apparently reduced neutropenia period in a limited number of radiation accident victims [13]. Waselenko and colleagues have recently presented recommended cytokine dosages.

Supportive care

Supportive care is essential for victims of moderate and higher levels of exposure (see Table 9). Care includes the use of cytokines, antimicrobials, blood components, antidiarrheal agents, fluids, electrolytes, analgesic agents, topical burn creams, and antiemetic agents. However, the early use of antiemetics may be impractical and even undesirable given the value of time of onset of vomiting as a factor in clinical dosimetry [13,39].

Prophylactic antibiotic therapy for exposures over 2 Gy should be initiated during the neutropenia period along with isolation for immunosuppression. Patients exhibiting absolute neutrophil count $<0.500 \times 10^9$ cells/L should receive broad-spectrum antimicrobial agents [38]. Recommended is fluoroquinolone with

Table 9
Principal therapeutic measures for acute radiation syndrome according to degree of severity

Whole body dose (Gy)	1–2	2–4	4–6	6–8	>8
Severity of ARS	Mild	Moderate	Severe	Very severe	Lethal
Medical management and treatment	Outpatient observation for maximum of 1 month	Hospitalization Isolation, as early as possible G-CSF or GM-CSF as early as possible (or within week 1) Antibiotics of broad spectrum activity (from the end of the latent period) Antifungal and antiviral preparations (when necessary) Blood components transfusion: platelets, erythrocytes (when necessary)	IL-3 and GM-CSF Complete parenteral nutrition (week 1) Metabolism correction, detoxification (when necessary) Plasmapheresis (week 2 or 3) Prophylaxis of disseminated intravascular coagulation (week 2)	HLA-identical allogene bone marrow transplantation (BMT) (week 1)	Symptomatic therapy only

Adapted from reference International Atomic Energy Agency. Diagnosis and treatment of radiation injuries. Safety Reports Series No. 2. Vienna: IAEA; 1998.

streptococcal coverage. If no streptococcal coverage, the fluoroquinolone should be administered with penicillin or amoxicillin. Prophylaxis with antifungal agents and antiviral agents for herpes simplex positive patients should be administered as appropriate. Antimicrobial therapy is continued until absolute neutrophil count is $\geq 0.500 \times 10^9$ cells/L, or it is clear the therapy is not effective. Additional guidelines on the effective use of antimicrobials are available [13].

The use of blood products to combat radiation-induced aplasia is normally not required for 2–4 weeks, allowing time for donors to be identified. Blood components should be leukoreduced and irradiated to prevent transfusion-associated, graft-versus-host disease in the immunosuppressed victim. The latter can be difficult to differentiate from organ toxicities exhibited during ARS [38].

Consideration of hematopoietic stem cell transplantation (SCT) requires early consultation with specialists uniquely familiar with the associated barriers [38]. Experience with past accidents has revealed that SCT has several limitations [10,13,38]. SCT should only be considered for victims receiving uniformly distributed doses of 7–10 Gy, exhibiting no significant burns, and minimal internal contamination. Early marrow transplantation is favored and reliable physical and biological dosimetry is essential.

Internal contamination treatment

Several excellent sources of information are available regarding the treatment of patients with internal radioisotope contamination [14,34,40]. The basic treatment principles are dilution, blocking, chelation, mobilization, and elimination of contaminant.

Gastric lavage and emetics can be used to empty the stomach, while purgatives, laxatives, and enemas reduce the residence time of the contaminant in the colon. In addition, Prussian blue has been found to be effective at increasing the removal rate of cesium, thallium, and rubidium by way of feces. Phosphates may be used to reduce the intestinal uptake of strontium. The most commonly known blocking agent, potassium iodide (KI), is valuable for prevention of radioiodine uptake by the thryroid. Common chelating agents are calcium and zinc diethylenetriaminepentaacetic acid, CaDTPA and ZnDTPA, respectively. These two agents form soluble complexes with americium and plutonium, as well as a number of rare earth, transition, and other transuranium metals, although they are only approved for the transuraniums.

Lung lavage has been used successfully in experimental animal studies for removing insoluble radioactive particles. Application in humans should be limited to alpha-emitting radioisotopes of significant activity [34].

Potassium Iodide

Administration of KI prophylaxis is restricted to scenarios involving fission radionuclide products from a nuclear detonation or a nuclear power-plant incident. Administration of KI for thyroid protection should occur immediately (<6 hours) post incident. Dosage guidance is available on the Centers for Disease Control and Prevention website at: www.bt.cdc.gov/radiation/ki.asp.

Combined injury treatment

A nuclear detonation or a major power-plant incident will expose victims to high levels of radiation and also result in thermal and radiation burns, wounds, fractures, or other trauma injuries. Such combined injuries can substantially worsen the prognosis of the patient. These victims may be predisposed to lethal infections caused by reduced immune function. This was observed for Chernobyl firefighters and should receive highest priority in the treatment of these individuals [32]. Lung damage from inhalation of radioactive particles could also result in tissue damage, edema, and pneumonia. Cutaneous syndrome involving damage to the skin, muscle, connective tissues, bone, and other tissues may require multiple surgeries to remove necrotic and infected tissue. Careful decontamination and debridement may substantially improve the prognosis of these local radiation injuries [5].

Radiation exposures involving children

Children require special consideration in the event of a radiologic incident [41]. Vulnerabilities include greater potential for internal exposure, increased likelihood of psychologic injury, potentially higher stochastic effects, and a wide range of identifiable abnormalities in utero. Neuropathology always accompanies in utero abnormalities because of the sensitivity of the developing neural system. Guidelines for the management of internally and externally exposed pregnant women and children are available [13,41]. A prenatal radiation exposure fact sheet is available at www.bt.cdc.gov/radiation/prenatalphysician.asp.

Summary

Many resources exist to assist emergency medicine and critical care physicians if presented with irradiated patients. Most knowledge has been gained caring for victims of accidents and nuclear detonation. Over the past 60 years, dose-dependent symptoms and symptom sequence have been established for a number of radiation-induced syndromes. However, early diagnosis in the absence of knowledge of radiation exposure can be a challenge for the clinician because of the nonspecific nature of symptoms. Diagnosis is greatly aided by use of biological dosimetry combining early emesis, lymphocyte depletion kinetics, and peripheral blood lymphocyte dicentrics. Biodosimetry is also a useful tool to assist with selection of therapeutic measures for externally and internally exposed victims, including those with combined injuries.

References

[1] Radiation Emergency Assistance Center/Training Site (REAC/TS). Accident statistics available by direct request. Available at: http://www.orau.gov/reacts. Accessed March 15, 2005.

[2] Spector M. Russians assert radioactive box found in park posed no danger. The New York Times November 25,1995;section A:5.

[3] Gertz B. Al Qaida pursued a dirty bomb. Nation/Politics section. The Washington Times October 16, 2003.

[4] Leikin JB, McFee RB, Walter FG, et al. A primer for nuclear terrorism. Dis Mon 2003;49: 479–516.

[5] National Council on Radiation Protection and Measurements. In: O'Brian CL, editor. Management of terrorist events involving radioactive material, No. 138. Bethesda (MD): NCRP; 2001. p. 1–4.

[6] Zimmerman PD. Dirty bombs: the threat revisited. Def Hor 2004;38:1–11.

[7] International Atomic Energy Agency. The radiological accident in Gioania. Safety reports series no. 2. Vienna: IAEA; 1988.

[8] Dowd S, Tilson E. Practical radiation protection and applied radiobiology. 2nd edition. Philadelphia: WB Saunders Co; 1999.

[9] United Nations. Sources and effects of ionizing radiation. Vol. II: effects. United Nations Scientific Committee on the Effects of Atomic Radiation. 2000 report to the General Assembly. United Nations # E.00.IX.4.

[10] International Atomic Energy Agency. Diagonosis and treatment of radiation injuries. Safety reports series no. 2. Vienna: IAEA; 1998.

[11] Guskova AK, Baranov AE, Gusev IA. Acute radiation sickness: underlying principles and assessment. In: Gusev IA, Guskova AK, Mettler FA, editors. Medical management of radiation accidents. 2nd edition. Orlando (FL): CRC Press; 2001. p. 33–51.

[12] The Illinois Emergency Management Agency. Radiation accidents: at the hospital. Available at: http://www.state.il.us/idns/pdfs/pubPDF/IEMA%20059.pdf. Accessed March 15, 2005.

[13] Waselenko JK, MacVittie TJ, Blakely WF, et al. Medical management of the acute radiation syndrome: recommendations of the strategic national stockpile radiation working group. Ann Intern Med 2004;140(12):1037–51.

[14] Armed Forces Radiobiology Research Institute. Medical management of radiological casualties – handbook. 2nd edition. Bethesda (MD): AFRRI; 2003.

[15] Mettler FA, Guskova AK. Treatment of acute radiation sickness. In: Gusev IA, Guskova AK, Mettler FA, editors. Medical management of radiation accidents. 2nd edition. Orlando (FL): CRC Press; 2001. p. 53–67.

[16] Gongora R, Magdelinar H. Accidental acute local irradiations in France and their pathology. Br J Radiol 1986;19:12–5.

[17] Barabanova A, Osanov DP. The dependence of skin lesions on the depth-dose distribution from β-irradiation of people in the Chernobyl nuclear power plant accident. Int J Radiat Biol 1990; 57(4):775–82.

[18] Barahanova AV. Local radiation injury. In: Gusev IA, Guskova AK, Mettler FA, editors. Medical management of radiation accidents. 2nd edition. Orlando (FL): CRC Press; 2001. p. 223–40.

[19] Barabanova AV. Acute radiation syndrome with cutaneous syndrome. In: Ricks RC, Berger ME, O'Hara FM, editors. The medical basis for radiation-accident preparedness: the clinical care of victims. New York: Parthenon; 2002. p. 217–24.

[20] Peter RU. Management of skin injuries in radiation accidents: the cutaneous radiation syndrome. In: Ricks RC, Berger ME, O'Hara RM, editors. The medical basis for radiation-accident preparedness: the clinical care of victims. New York: Parthenon; 2002. p. 225–9.

[21] Smith JM, Fong F. Clinician briefing: radiation emergencies. Available at: http://www.bt.cdc. gov/coca/summaries/radiation022404.asp. Accessed March 15, 2005.

[22] Oak Ridge Associated Universities. Managing radiation emergencies: guidance for hospital medical management. Available at: http://www.orau.gov/reacts/syndrome.htm. Accessed March 15, 2005.

[23] Brodsky A. Radioactivity hazards in survival planning. American Academy health physics course 1: materials and methods for training responders to radiation emergencies. January 25, 2003.

[24] Anderson V. Radiological dispersion devices – A.K.A. "the dirty bomb." Presented at the 36th Annual Midyear Meeting of the Health Physics Society. San Antonio, Texas, January 26–29, 2003.

[25] Behrens C, Holt M. Nuclear power plants: vulnerability to terrorist attack. Available at: http://www.fas.org/irp/crs/RS21131.pdf. Accessed March 1, 2005.

[26] Department of Homeland Security. Medical preparedness response sub-group. Available at: http://www.va.gov/emshg/docs/Radiologic_Medical_Countermeasures_051403.pdf. Accessed March 15, 2005.

[27] Kearsley EE. Health physics society educational briefing. Radiologial terrorism: Dirty bombs – fact and fiction. April 8, 2003. Available to members at http://www.hps.org/searchresult.cfm. Accessed March 15, 2005.

[28] Shea DA. Radiological dispersal devices: select issues in consequence management. Available at: http://www.law.umaryland.edu/marshall/crsreports/crsdocuments/RS21766_03102004.pdf. Accessed March 1, 2005.

[29] Howe D. Planning scenarios – executive summaries. Available at: http://www.globalsecurity.org/ security/library/report/2004/hsc-planning-scenarios-jul04.htm. Accessed March 1, 2005.

[30] Mettler FA. Emergency room management of radiation incidents. In: Gusev IA, Guskova AK, Mettler FA, editors. Medical management of radiation accidents. 2nd edition. Orlando (FL): CRC Press; 2001. p. 437–47.

[31] Dainiak N. Hematologic consequences of exposure to ionizing radiation. Exp Hematol 2002;30: 513–28.

[32] National Council on Radiation Protection and Measurement. Medical Management of Radiation Casualties. In: O'Brian CL, editor. Management of terrorist events involving radioactive material. No. 138. Bethesda (MD): NCRP; 2001. p. 27–69.

[33] Mettler FA. Hospital preparation for radiation accidents. In: Gusev IA, Guskova AK, Mettler FA, editors. Medical management of radiation accidents. 2nd edition. Orlando (FL): CRC Press; 2001. p. 425–35.

[34] Voelz GL. Assessment and treatment of internal contamination: general principles. In: Gusev IA, Guskova AK, Mettler FA, editors. Medical management of radiation accidents. 2nd edition. Orlando (FL): CRC Press; 2001. p. 319–36.

[35] Bender MA, Gooch PC. Somatic chromosome aberrations induced by human whole-body irradiation: the "Recuplex" criticality accident. Radiat Res 1966;29:568–82.

[36] Koteles GJ, Benko I. Thermography in radiation injuries. Thermolog Osten 1994;4:55–65.

[37] Nenot JC. Medical and surgical management for localized radiation injuries. Int J Radiat Biol 1990;57:783–95.

[38] Dainiak N, Waselenlso JK, Armitage JO, et al. The hematologist and radiation casualties. Hematol 2003;1:473–95 Available at: http://www.asheducationbook.org/cgi/content/full/2003/1/ 473. Accessed March 15, 2005.

[39] Goans RE. Clinical care of the radiation-accident patient: patient presentation, assessment, and initial diagnosis. In: Ricks RC, Berger ME, O'Hara FM, editors. The medical basis for radiation-accident preparedness. the clinical-care of victims. New York: Parthenon; 2002. p. 11–22.

[40] National Council on Radiation Protection and Measurement. Management of persons accidently contaminated with radionuclides. No. 65. Bethesda (MD): NCRP; 1980.

[41] American Academy of Pediatrics. Policy statement: radiation disasters and children. Pediatrics 2003;111(6):1455–66.

ELSEVIER
SAUNDERS

Crit Care Clin 21 (2005) 815–824

CRITICAL
CARE
CLINICS

Ricin

Laura Spivak, MD*, Robert G. Hendrickson, MD

*Department of Emergency Medicine, Oregon Health and Science University,
3181 SW Sam Jackson Park Road, Portland, OR 97239, USA*

Ricin, a potent toxin contained in the beans of the castor plant (*Ricinus communis*), has a colorful history. The plant originated in Asia and Africa and can now be found in all temperate and subtropical regions [1]. The innocuous appearing castor plant grows wild across the southwestern United States and is cultivated for decorative purposes [2]. Within its black and brown seeds is the glycoprotein ricin, which makes up 1% to 5% of the weight of the castor bean [3,4]. Another extract from the beans, castor oil, is non-toxic, contains no ricin, and has been used for centuries as a laxative, lubricating oil (eg, Castrol-R racing motor oil), and paint and varnish additive [1,2,4]. Castor oil was used by the military as an aircraft lubricant from World War I though the 1960s [2].

Although ricin was first perceived as a biological warfare agent during World War I, it has more recently been identified as an agent that may be used by terrorists against civilians [1,2,5]. Ricin is one of the most potent plant toxins known [2]. It is much easier to produce than other biological agents, such as anthrax or botulinum toxin [2,4]; production requires only basic techniques that are taught in undergraduate-level chemistry classes [6,7]. The potency of ricin, and the ease with which it can be produced, likely explain why it is frequently associated with extremist individuals and terrorist organizations [3].

In the 1920s, several nations, including the United States, began research on the use of ricin as a biological warfare agent [1,3]. In the United States, ricin was given the code name "Compound W" [1,3]. During World War II, the United States and Great Britain collaborated on the production of a bomb that contained ricin [2,3]; however, although this "W bomb" underwent testing, it

---

* Corresponding author.
E-mail address: spivakl@ohsu.edu (L. Spivak).

0749-0704/05/$ – see front matter © 2005 Elsevier Inc. All rights reserved.
doi:10.1016/j.ccc.2005.06.006   *criticalcare.theclinics.com*

was never used in combat [3]. After World War II, the United States and the Soviet Union continued to study ricin as a weapon, and in 1989, the Iraqi government allegedly tested the use of aerosolized ricin [2].

Ricin was also used as a homicidal agent by the Soviet Komitet Gosudarstvennoi Bezopasnosti (KGB). In 1978, a Bulgarian exile named Georgi Markov was assassinated in London. The assassin used a spring-loaded needle mounted within an umbrella to inject a small pellet of ricin into Mr. Markov's thigh [3]. He developed constitutional symptoms within a day and died 4 days later [8]. Another attempted homicide involving ricin occurred one month before this attack. Vladimir Kostov, a Bulgarian state radio and television correspondent, sustained a blow to his back in a Paris metro station. He was hospitalized for 12 days with a fever. After reading about the Markov case he was re-examined by physicians and the same type of ricin bullet was discovered in his skin. The bullet had not penetrated through the subcutaneous fat layer and so no ricin was absorbed systemically [1,8].

Since the 1990s, ricin has been found during seizure and examination of terrorist-related communications and documents [3,4]. In January 2003, authorities arrested six men suspected of producing ricin in their North London apartment [9,10]. In October 2003, a threatening letter along with a sealed container of ricin was processed at a mail facility in Greenville, South Carolina. The author threatened to poison the water supply if his demands were not met [11]. In January 2005, a 22-year-old man was arrested in Ocala, Florida, after a box of ricin was found in his home [12]. In February 2004, ricin powder was discovered on a mail-sorting machine in United States Senator Bill Frist's office building. Plans for ricin production were discovered in the possession of Chechen rebels and in Kabul, Afghanistan; both circumstances were thought to be related to planned terrorist activity [4].

Mechanism of toxicity

The toxicity of ricin is dependent on both the dose delivered and the route of the exposure [3,13]. The median lethal dose (LD_{50}) is the dose that would kill 50% of the people to whom it was applied; the smaller the LD_{50}, the less material is needed to kill the average person. For ricin, the LD_{50} is lowest for inhalation, and increases respectively for intravenous, intraperitoneal, subcutaneous, and intragastric administration [3]. Aerosolized ricin may lead to local pulmonary effects [14] as well as systemic effects following absorption. Ingestion of ricin is less likely to lead to toxicity, because of poor gastrointestinal absorption and potential enzymatic degradation of the protein within the gastrointestinal tract [3]. Contact allergies have been reported from dermal exposure (castor bean necklaces) [15]. Dermal absorption of ricin is poor [3,13], but systemic toxicity is possible if ricin is mixed in a solvent liquid, such as dimethyl sulfoxide [4], and is dispersed as an aerosol or liquid.

Ricin is a Type II ribosome-inactivating protein [1,2], which consists of two polypeptide chains bridged by a disulfide bond [1,2]. These chains must be linked to cause toxicity [1,3]. The B-chain, a lectin, has galactose-binding sites on either end to facilitate hydrogen bonding with cell surface glycoproteins and glycolipids [1,2,16,17]. The A-chain is an N-glycosidase [18,19] that removes adenine from the 28 S ribosomal RNA subunit [19]. This halts the binding of elongation factors, which results in the failure of protein synthesis [18,20]. Ricin is internalized by way of multiple mechanisms, including receptor-mediated endocytosis (Fig. 1) [21]. It is initially transported to the Golgi apparatus, then

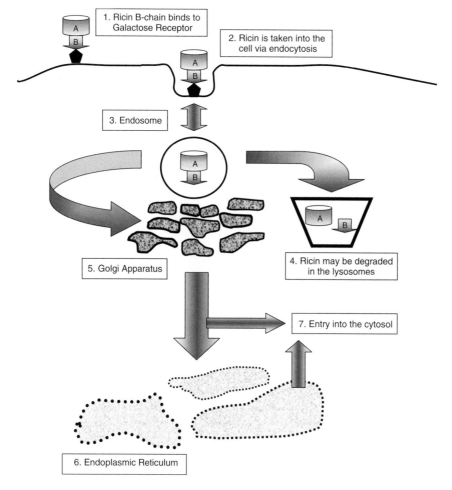

Fig. 1. Possible mechanisms of ricin entry into the cytosol. Steps in ricin internalization: The ricin B-chain binds to galactose receptors on the cell surface (1), and is endocytosed (2) into an endosome (3). Ricin is then either degraded by lysosomes (4) or transported into the Golgi apparatus (5), then either transported directly into the cytosol, or to the endoplasmic reticulum (6), and then into the cytosol (7).

the endoplasmic reticulum, and finally translocated to the cytosol [2,17,22]. Delivery to intracellular compartments is relatively slow (10% per hour at 37°C) [1,23]; however, only a small number of molecules present in the cytosol are necessary to produce cell death [2,18,24,25].

Ricin's potential as an immunotoxin has been studied since 1951, when the A-chain was discovered to inhibit tumor growth [1]. It has been used in Phase I and II clinical trials alone or as a component of tumor cell-specific antibodies (immunotoxins) [26–28]. Vascular leak syndrome, the result of ricin-mediated endothelial cell destruction, is a dose-limiting side effect resulting in hypoalbuminemia and edema [28]. Other limitations of therapy include the antibody's lack of specificity, and the immunogenicity of the toxin, which creates a refractory immunity in the host [27]. This immunogenicity has been exploited in the hopes of developing a ricin vaccine [29].

Clinical presentation

Ricin inhibits protein synthesis diffusely, and its systemic manifestations are non-specific and widespread. Signs and symptoms from oral and parenteral exposures resemble diffuse endothelial damage or the Systemic Inflammatory Response Syndrome (SIRS), and include fever, tachycardia, tachypnea, hypotension, hepatitis, pancreatitis, nephritis, myocardial injury, cerebral edema, vomiting, diarrhea, and bone marrow suppression [2,3,13]. The onset of symptoms after an exposure to ricin may be delayed for several hours. In vivo, the latency period between exposure and the symptom onset ranges from 8 to 24 hours [3]. Reports of non-fatal ingestions have demonstrated symptoms manifesting within several hours after ingestion [30–33]. Documented fatal and non-fatal human exposures have reported nausea, vomiting, abdominal cramps, diarrhea, dehydration, gastrointestinal hemorrhage, anuria, mydriasis, fever, and hypotension [2,3,13,30–34]. Transaminitis is commonly seen in patients [13] and may develop several days after the exposure [34]. In severe cases, death may ensue within several days [3], or patients may require several weeks of intensive care.

The only human data available for inhalational ricin exposure involves workers exposed to castor bean dust in castor oil processing plants. These patients developed nasal and throat congestion, irritation of the conjunctivae, urticaria, chest tightness, and bronchospasm [35]. Removal from exposure and supportive care led to symptom resolution [36]. Immunohistochemical studies in rats exposed to aerosolized ricin show that ricin binds to ciliated bronchiolar lining cells, alveolar macrophages, and alveolar lining cells [3]. A diffuse, necrotizing pneumonia, with interstitial and alveolar inflammation and edema, was observed in rats 8 hours after inhaling lethal doses of ricin [3]. A primate study found a dose-dependent latency period of 8 to 24 hours following ricin inhalation, followed by the onset of anorexia, decreased physical activity, and death within 36–48 hours. The time to death was also dose-dependent [3]. Acute tracheitis, airway inflammation and necrosis, diffuse alveolar flooding, fibrino-purulent pneumonia, and purulent mediastinal lymphadenitis were seen on necropsy [37].

Although orally ingested ricin may lead to nausea, vomiting, diarrhea, dehy-dration, gastrointestinal hemorrhage, and hypotension, ingestion of intact castor beans rarely results in systemic symptoms or death. In fact, from 1983 to 2002, no deaths from castor bean exposure were reported to the American Association of Poison Control Centers Toxic Exposure Surveillance System [38], and there have been no reported fatalities from castor bean ingestion since 1935 [2].

When orally ingested, ricin acts locally on the intestinal mucosa, and ex-cess toxin may be enzymatically degraded [39]. Mastication of castor beans may facilitate ricin release and increase the risk of local or systemic toxicity [13]. Autopsy findings following ingestion include hemorrhage and ulceration within the gastric and small-intestinal mucosa, necrosis of mesenteric lymph nodes, hepatic necrosis, as well as nephritis and splenitis. Once absorbed, ricin con-centrates within the liver and spleen [39,40], possibly because of the presence of mannose receptors on the cells of the reticuloendothelial system (Kupffer cells and macrophages), which render them vulnerable to binding of the B-chain [13].

Parenteral ricin, when used in clinical trials in doses up to 23 mcg/m^2, has been well tolerated [26]. Fatigue and muscle pain were reported within 4 to 6 hours of the injections and these symptoms lasted for 24–48 hours [41]. Rats demonstrated Kupffer cell damage within 4 hours of being given intravenous ricin. Subsequent hepatic thrombi with resultant hepatocellular necrosis oc-curred after damage to the sinusoidal cells [42,43]. A transient leukocytosis in humans has been seen with both oral and intravenous administration of ricin [3]. There is a twofold to fivefold increase in the leukocyte count observed in cancer patients receiving ricin therapy [3,8]. Disseminated intravascular coagu-lation is seen in experimental animals that have received high-dose intravenous ricin [3]. Resultant hepatic and renal injuries may be secondary to toxin-mediated vascular damage and not direct toxin-mediated effects [44].

Intramuscular and subcutaneous injections of high doses of ricin in humans result in localized pain within the soft tissues and regional lymphadenitis [8]. Georgi Markov, the assassinated Bulgarian exile, received an estimated 500 μg of ricin injected into his right thigh. He developed immediate pain at the injection site, and complained of weakness within 5 hours of the injection [3]. He became febrile within 24 hours, with nausea and vomiting. He was not admitted to a hospital until 36 hours later, at which time he experienced fever, tachycardia, a stable blood pressure, and inguinal lymphadenopathy ipsilateral to the injection site. He developed induration around the puncture site. Approximately 48 hours after the injection, he became hypotensive and tachycardic (160 beats per minute). His white blood cell count was 26,300/mm^3. By the third day he had developed hematemesis and anuria. On the fourth day after the injection, he developed atrioventricular dissociation, cardiac arrest, and died. His final white blood cell count was 33,200/mm^3 [8]. A 36-year-old man injected the contents of a single castor bean (approximately 150 mg of ricin) intramuscularly and developed headache, rigors, nausea, and tachycardia, with erythema and lymph-adenopathy local to the injection site [45]. A 20-year-old man injected the extracted liquid of castor beans subcutaneously and developed abdominal pain, myalgias, vomiting, hypotension, metabolic acidosis, gastrointestinal bleeding, anuria, and death within several days of the injection [46].

Impact on critical care

Exposure to ricin may produce victims that require critical care in several ways. The contamination of communal resources, such as the food and water supply, could lead to a large number of exposures across widespread geographic areas with simultaneous presentations. Although it is likely that only a small percentage of these victims would require critical care, this may equate to a relatively large absolute number of critically ill patients. Alternatively, a small number of people may be targeted and poisoned by way of food or water supplies. This scenario may be more difficult to detect as the symptomatology is typically non-specific and may be confused with several other terrorist agents and naturally occurring diseases (Box 1). Finally, aerosolized ricin has the potential to expose a large number of people to a significant quantity of ricin at the same time. Patients may require critical care because of pulmonary edema and necrosis as well as systemic toxicity.

Box 1. Differential diagnosis

Staphylococcal enterotoxin B [3,5]
Tricothecene mycotoxin
Pyrolysis byproducts of Teflon, Kevlar (DuPont) [3]
Phosgene [3,5]
Paraquat [3]
Biologic toxins (*Staphylococcus aureus*, salmonella, shigella)
Viruses (Influenza, Norwalk virus, Rotavirus, Adenovirus)
Systemic Inflammatory Response Syndrome or Sepsis
Tularemia [5]
Plague [5]
Acute arsenic toxicity
Acute inorganic mercury, thallium, or iron ingestion
Acute radiation sickness
Chemotherapeutic agents
Capillary leak syndromes–autoimmune vasculitis, SJS

Decontamination

Patients who are exposed to ricin by way of liquid, powder, or aerosol must have their clothing removed and their skin thoroughly washed for 5–6 minutes with water before admission to the hospital [47]. Ricin does not require any unique external decontamination techniques [5].

If the patient was exposed by way of the gastrointestinal tract, or the exposure is unknown, gastrointestinal decontamination with gastric lavage and activated charcoal may be appropriate; however, gastric lavage is not likely to remove a significant amount of ricin unless it is performed within 1 hour of ingestion [48]. Ricin is poorly adsorbed by activated charcoal because of its large size [5]; however, activated charcoal may adsorb a small fraction of available ricin in the gastrointestinal tract and prevent absorption. Once absorbed, elimination techniques, including hemodialysis, are not effective. Once the patient has been externally decontaminated, they do not require isolation, negative pressure, or any personal protective equipment other than universal precautions [5,14]. Vomitus and diarrhea should be handled with barrier and splash precautions (eg, gown, eyeshield, mask, gloves), but is unlikely to produce a vapor or to expose health care workers to contamination [5].

Diagnostic studies

Laboratory evaluation should include renal and liver function tests, and electrolytes, which may need repletion secondary to volume loss. Critically ill and hypotensive patients should be evaluated with laboratory tests as if they have SIRS or sepsis, including blood gas, lactate, electrolyte panel including renal function tests, complete blood count, blood cultures, and cortisol testing.

Ricin may be detected via radioimmunoassay, ELISA, polymerase chain reaction (PCR), ricinine detection protocol, and time-resolved fluorescence immunoassay (TRF) [2]. Ricin has been measured in very low concentrations in both serum (1.5 µg/L) and urine (0.3 µg/L) after poisoning [32]. ELISA can detect ricin in human urine and serum at concentrations as low as 100 pg/mL [49]. This method is safe and accurate for use in the clinical setting [2]. Clinical testing for ricin may be performed by PCR at a regional public health laboratory by collecting 25 mL of urine [50,51]. The urine should be packaged as is instructed by the Centers for Disease Control and Prevention (www.bt. cdc.gov/labissues/pdf/shipping-samples.pdf and www.bt.cdc.gov/labissues/pdf/ chemspecimencollection.pdf) [50,51]. TRF is a qualitative assay involving ricin-binding antibodies. It takes approximately 4 hours to complete. Faster assays will be required to detect aerosolized ricin [2]. To date, lab findings in animals exposed to airborne ricin are non-specific [3]. Antibodies are not detectable on initial evaluation; however, they may be present 2 weeks after exposure. [3] Early studies in rabbits and mice showed that these antibodies cross the placenta and are excreted in breast milk [3].

Antidotes, treatment, and supportive care

Supportive care is the mainstay of treatment. Hypotension should be treated with aggressive fluid replacement and direct-acting vasopressors, including phenylephrine, epinephrine, norepinephrine, or vasopressin. There is no evidence that any individual pressor is superior to another. However, there is evidence of increased endogenous norepinephrine release following ricin administration in rabbits, as well as decreased vascular responsiveness to norepinephrine [52,53]. Given this, vasopressin may be a reasonable alternative if catecholamines are ineffective.

Patients with non-cardiogenic pulmonary edema or airway edema may require mechanical ventilation. Although there is no research available to guide ventilator strategies, the pathophysiology of ricin pulmonary toxicity is a diffuse, inflammatory cellular toxicity. Therefore, ventilation strategies should likely mimic those for chemical pneumonitis or Acute Respiratory Distress Syndrome, with low tidal volume ventilation as a reasonable starting point [54].

Summary

Although ricin's history as a biologic weapon consists only of discrete episodes of poisoning, its widespread availability and ease of manufacture make it a viable terrorist threat. Clinicians must maintain a low threshold of suspicion for patients presenting with non-specific systemic illnesses, and be especially vigilant regarding large numbers of patients exhibiting gastrointestinal or pulmonary symptoms. The authors have outlined a plan of supportive care and diagnostic testing, that, along with a comprehensive differential diagnosis, should aid physicians in diagnosing and treating terrorist incidents involving ricin.

References

[1] Olsnes S. The history of ricin, abrin, and related toxins. Toxicon 2004;44:361–70.
[2] Doan LG. Ricin: mechanism of toxicity, clinical manifestations, and vaccine development. A review. J Toxicol Clin Toxicol 2004;42:201–8.
[3] Franz DR, Jaax NK. Ricin toxin. In: Sidell FR, Takafuji ET, Franz DR, editors. Medical aspects of chemical and biological warfare. Washington (DC): Office of the Surgeon General/TMM publications; 1997. p. 631–42.
[4] Henghold W. Other biologic toxin bioweapons: ricin, staphylococcal enterotoxin B, and trichothecene mycotoxins. Dermatol Clin 2004;22:257–62.
[5] Ricin. In: Kortepeter M, Christopher G, Cieslak T, et al, editors. USAMRIID's medical management of biological casualties handbook. 4th edition. Frederick (MD): United States Army Medical Research Institute of Infectious Disease; 2001. p. 130–7.
[6] Darby S, Miller M, Allen R. Forensic determination of ricin and the alkaloid marker ricinine from castor bean extracts. J Forensic Sci 2001;46:1033–42.
[7] Marks J. Medical aspects of biologic toxins. Anesthesiology Clin N Am 2004;22:509–32.

[8] Crompton R, Gall D. Georgi Markov: death in a pellet. Med Leg J 1980;48:51–62.

[9] Bale J, Bhattacharjee A, Croddy E, et al. Ricin found in London: an al-Qa'ida connection?: CNS Reports. Available at: www.cns.miis.edu/pubs/reports/ricin.htm. Accessed February 9, 2005.

[10] Mayor S. UK doctors warned after ricin poison found in police raid. BMJ 2003;326:126.

[11] Investigation of a ricin-containing envelope at a postal facility - South Carolina. MMWR 2003; 52:1129–31.

[12] Associated_Press. Man arrested after ricin found in home. Available at: www.foxnews.com. Accessed February 9, 2005.

[13] Bradberry S, Dickers K, Rice P, et al. Ricin poisoning. Toxicol Rev 2003;22:65–70.

[14] Bunner D. Biological warfare agents: an overview. In: Somani S, editor. Chemical warfare agents. San Diego (CA): Academic Press; 1992. p. 387.

[15] Schaumburg H, Spencer P. Ricin. In: Spencer P, Schaumberg H, editors. Experimental and clinical neurotoxicology. 2nd edition. New York: Oxford University Press; 2000. p. 1068–9.

[16] Wales R, Richardson P, Roberts L, et al. Mutational analysis of the galactose binding ability of recombinant ricin B chain. J Biol Chem 1991;266:19172–9.

[17] Sandvig K, van Deurs B. Transport of protein toxins into cells: pathways used by ricin, cholera toxin and Shiga toxin. FEBS Lett 2002;529:49–53.

[18] Endo Y, Mitsui K, Motizuki MKT. The mechanism of action of ricin and related toxic lectins on eukaryotic ribosomes. The site and the characteristics of the modification in 28s ribosomal rna caused by the toxins. J Biol Chem 1987;262:5908–12.

[19] Endo Y, Tsurugi K. RNA N-glycosidase activity of ricin a-chain. Mechanism of action of the toxic lectin ricin on eukaryotic ribosomes. J Biol Chem 1987;262:8128–30.

[20] Olsnes S. Closing in on ricin action. Nature 1987;328:474–5.

[21] Lord MJ, Jolliffe NA, Marsden CJ, et al. Ricin: mechanisms of cytotoxicity. Toxicol Rev 2003;22:53–64.

[22] Sandvig K, Grimmer S, Lauvrak S, et al. Pathways followed by ricin and Shiga toxin into cells. Histochem Cell Biol 2002;117:131–41.

[23] Montanaro L, Sperti S, Stirpe F. Inhibition by ricin of protein synthesis in vitro. Ribosomes as the target of the toxin. Biochem J 1973;136:677–83.

[24] Wiley R, Oeltmann T. Ricin and related plant toxins: mechanism of action and neurobiological applications. In: Keeler R, Tu A, editors. Toxicology of plant and fungal compounds. New York: Marcel Dekker; 1991. p. 243.

[25] Eiklid K, Olsnes S, Pihl A. Entry of lethal doses of abrin, ricin, and modeccin into the ecytosol of HeLa cells. Exp Cell Res 1980;126:321–6.

[26] Fodstad O, Kvalheim G, Godal A, et al. Phase I study of the plant protein ricin. Cancer Res 1984;44:862–5.

[27] Vitetta E, Krolick K, Muneo M, et al. Immunotoxins: a new approach to cancer therapy. Science 1983;219:644–9.

[28] Soler-Rodriguez A, Ghetie M, Oppenheimer-Marks N, et al. Ricin A-chain and ricin A-chain immunotoxins rapidly damage human endothelial cells: implications for vascular leak syndrome. Exp Cell Res 1993;206:227–34.

[29] Smallshaw J, Firan A, Fulmer J, et al. A novel recombinant vaccine which protects mice against ricin intoxication. Vaccine 2002;20:3422–77.

[30] Palatnick W, Tenenbein M. Hepatotoxicity from castor bean ingestion in a child. Clin Toxicol 2000;38:67–9.

[31] Rauber A, Heard J. Castor bean toxicity re-examined: a new perspective. Vet Hum Toxicol 1985;27:498–502.

[32] Kopferschmitt J, Flesch F, Lugnier A, et al. Acute voluntary intoxication by ricin. Hum Toxicol 1983;2:239–42.

[33] Aplin P, Eliseo T. Ingestion of castor oil plant seeds. Med J Aust 1997;167:260–1.

[34] Levin Y, Sherer Y, Bibi H, et al. Rare Jatropha multifida intoxication in two children. J Emerg Med 2000;19:173–5.

[35] Topping M, Henderson R, Luczynska C, et al. Castor bean allergy among workers in the felt industry. Allergy 1982;37:603–8.

[36] Brugsch H. Toxic hazards: the castor bean. Mass Med Soc 1960;262:1039–40.

[37] Wilhelmsen C, Pitt L. Lesions of acute inhaled lethal ricin intoxication in rhesus monkeys. Vet Pathol 1993;30:482.

[38] Watson W, Litovitz T, Rodgers GJ, et al. 2002 annual report of the american association of poison control centers toxic exposure surveillance system. Am J Emerg Med 2003;21:353–421.

[39] Fodstad O, Olsnes S, Pihl A. Toxicity, distribution and elimination of the cancerostatic lectins abrin and ricin after parenteral injection into mice. Br J Cancer 1976;34:418–25.

[40] Ramsden C, Drayson M, Bell E. The toxicity, distribution, and excretion of ricin holotoxin in rats. Toxicology 1989;55:161–71.

[41] Lambert J, Goldmacher V, Collinson A, et al. An immunotoxin prepared with blocked ricin: a natural plant toxin adapted for therapeutic use. Cancer Res 1991;51:6236–44.

[42] Bingen A, Creppy E, Gut J, et al. The Kupffer cell is the first target in ricin-induced hepatitis. J Submicrosc Cytol 1987;19:247–56.

[43] Derenzini M, Bonetti E, Marionozzi V, et al. Toxic effects of ricin: studies on the pathogenesis of liver lesions. Virchows Arch B Cell Pathol 1976;20:15–28.

[44] Howat A. The toxic plant proteins ricin and abrin induce apoptotic changes in mammalian lymphoid tissues and intestine. J Pathol 1988;154:29–33.

[45] Fine D, Shepherd H, Grifffiths G. Sub-lethal poisoning by self-injection with ricin. Med Sci Law 1992;32(1):70–2.

[46] Targosz D, Winnik L, Szkolnicka B. Suicidal poisoning with castor bean (Ricinus communis) extract injected subcutaneously: case report [abstract]. J Toxicol Clin Toxicol 2002;40:398.

[47] OSHA. Practices for hospital-based first receivers of victims from mass casualty incidents involving the release of hazardous substances. Available at: www.osha.gov/dts/osta/bestpractices/firstreceivers_hospital.htm. Accessed July 26, 2005.

[48] Vale JA. Gastric Lavage [position statement]. J Clin Toxicol 1997;35:711–9.

[49] Poli M, Rivera V, Hewetson J, et al. Detection of ricin by colorimetric and chemiluminescence ELISA. Toxicon 1994;32:1371–7.

[50] Chemical terrorism event specimen collection. Available at: www.bt.cdc.gov/labissues/pdf/chemspecimencollection.pdf. Accessed July 26, 2005.

[51] Shipping instructions for specimens collected from people potentially exposed to chemical terrorism agents. Available at: www.bt.cdc.gov/labissues/pdf/shipping-samples.pdf. Accessed July 26, 2005.

[52] Christiansen VJ, Hsu C-H, Robinson CP. The effects of ricin on the sympathetic vascular neuroeffector system of the rabbit. J Biochem Toxicology 1994;9(4):219–23.

[53] Christiansen VJ, Hsu C-H, Zhang L, Robinson CP. Effects of ricin on the ability of rabbit arteries to contract and relax. Journal of Applied Toxicology 1995;15(1):37–43.

[54] Brower R, Matthay M, Morris A, et al. Ventilation with lower tidal volumes as compared with traditional tidal volumes for acute lung injury and the acute respiratory distress syndrome. N Engl J Med 2000;342:1301–8.

ELSEVIER
SAUNDERS

CRITICAL
CARE
CLINICS

Crit Care Clin 21 (2005) 825–839

Botulinum Toxin

B. Zane Horowitz, MD, FACMT

Oregon Health and Sciences University, 3181 SW Sam Jackson Park Road, Portland, OR 97239, USA

Botulinum toxin is regarded as the most lethal substance known, on a weight basis, with a known median lethal dose (LD_{50}) of 1 nanogram of toxin per kilogram body mass [1]. The LD_{50} is the dose of liquid that would kill 50% of the people to whom it was applied; the smaller the LD_{50}, the less material is needed to kill the average person. The bacteria *Clostridium botulinum* that produces the botulinum toxin is present in soil throughout the world, and may exist in both freshwater and coastal saltwater mud [2]. Despite its widespread accessibility and high lethality, the botulinum toxin has never been used successfully for purposes of warfare or bioterrorism.

Botulinum toxin was investigated as a biologic agent by the British, American, Canadian, Japanese, and Soviet military since World War II. During World War II, Japan's infamous Unit 731 experimented with botulism by feeding it to prisoners in Manchuria [1]. Botulism's sole link to a presumed successful planned use as a weapon is provided by Paul Fildes, a high-ranking British specialist in bacterial weapons development during World War II, who has alluded to the fact that he contributed to the assassination of Reinhard Heydrick, head of the Gestapo [3]. The British supplied the Czech underground with a modified hand grenade—made with an attached glass vial containing botulism—that was used in the ambush of Heydrick's car.

The Soviets have run tests exposing animals to botulinum toxin at their Vozrozhdeniye Island site in the Aral Sea [1]. In the early 1990s, before their attack with Sarin on the Tokyo subway system, the Japanese cult Aum Shinrikyo, had released an ineffectively produced *C botulinum* preparation in Japan, which targeted a US military installation. They also planned a release during the Japanese prince's wedding [1].

E-mail address: horowiza@ohsu.edu

During the United Nations' inspections of Iraq's capabilities for biologic warfare in 1991, after the first Gulf War, botulinum toxin was clearly an area in which research had been directed. More botulinum toxin was produced than any other weaponizable agent in Iraq. Approximately 19,000 L were produced, of which approximately half was loaded onto warheads [1,4]. When General Hussein Kamal Hassan defected from Iraq in August 1995, he verified that he was personally aware of 100 bombs, 13 SCUD/Al Hussein missiles, and 122 mm rockets that were loaded with botulinum toxin as part of Iraq's biologic weapons program [3,4].

A more recent event occurred in November 2004, when an osteopathic physician, (who had previously had his license revoked, but operated a cosmetic clinic in Florida) and his girlfriend were admitted to hospitals in New Jersey suffering from respiratory failure. A married couple (a chiropractor and his wife) who were treated at this physician's clinic were simultaneously hospitalized for weakness in Florida. Investigation of this event revealed that this physician purchased large quantities of research-grade botulinum toxin, not intended for human use. He then attempted to compound it on his own to a more dilute concentration equivalent to Botox. Commercial Botox was not involved. All four victims required mechanical ventilation for several months. It was confirmed that three of these cases were caused by botulinum toxin.

Mechanism of toxicity

Clostridium botulinum, and three other clostridial organisms, produce the botulinum toxin. There are eight known serotypes of botulism, designated A through G, and C-α and C-β subgroups [1,2,5–7]. Almost all human cases of botulism are caused by serotypes A, B, and E [5]. There is a geographic predilection by serotype: type A primarily occurs west of the Mississippi River and type B typically occurs along the eastern part of North America and in Europe [2]. Type E is associated with eating certain marine animals, especially when improperly stored, and has occurred most frequently in the Great Lakes region, in Alaska, Canada, and Scandinavia [2,5,8]. Occasional cases of type F elaborated by *C baratii* [9], and type E elaborated by *C butyricum* [10] have also been reported, and rare human cases of type C-α and D, which mostly occurs in ducks, have occurred. No human disease has been caused by type C-β or G (Table 1).

Table 1
Clostridium organisms and botulinum serotypes

Organism	Botulism serotype	Human disease
Clostridium botulinum	A, B, C, D, E, F	Yes
Clostridium baratii	E	Yes
Clostridium butyricum	F	Yes
Clostridium argentinense	G	No

Originally, three forms of disease had been recognized: food-borne, wound and infant intestinal botulism. More recently, three additional forms have been reported: undefined or adult intestinal, inadvertent injection-related, and inhalational botulism. These clinical presentations are described below.

Classic food-borne botulism occurs through the ingestion of improperly canned or preserved food, which allows the growth of *C botulinum,* and elaboration of spores [2,11,12]. Spores can be dormant, resistant to heat, and germinate in low acidity (pH > 4.5), low salinity (NaCl < 3.5%), and low nitrate environments [5]. Canned vegetables, items preserved in garlic oil, and soups are usually the cause of sporadic outbreaks [5,11–13].

Wound botulism occurs through colonization of wounds with *C botulinum* [14–21]. Post-surgical cases were initially the cause of wound botulism [14,15], but almost all recent cases involved contaminated heroin in injection drug users [16–21]. The wounds involved do not necessarily appear infected on inspection, but may still harbor the organism.

Infant (intestinal) botulism, now the most commonly reported form of the disease, occurs through infant ingestion of *C botulinum* spores [22–24]. An infant's immature gastrointestinal tract allows the spores to germinate and elaborate the botulinum toxin. Patients present with constipation, feeding difficulties, and poor muscle tone. Feeding honey to a child under the age of 1 has been linked to many, but not all, cases of infant (intestinal) botulism [25].

The Centers for Disease Control and Prevention (CDC) recognizes a fourth classification, which is officially called undefined botulism, but is also referred to as adult-type infant botulism [2,6]. This delayed-onset neurologic syndrome mainly occurs in adults with abnormal gastrointestinal pathology, such as peptic ulcer disease, Billroth surgery, or Crohn's disease.

Inadvertent (injection-related) botulism is a fifth category associated with therapeutic misadventures from injection of pharmaceutical botulinum toxin [26]. Both Botox (botulinum type A toxin) and Myobloc (botulinum type B toxin) are available to treat a variety of spastic myopathies, and for treatment of glabelar lines (wrinkles).

However, there is concern over a new sixth category, inhalational botulism, which would only occur through the deliberate release of the botulinum toxin [1]. It is estimated that the human LD_{50} for inhalation botulism is 1 to 3 ng/kg [1]. To date only a single incident in three laboratory workers has been described.

The botulinum toxin, once elaborated in the gastrointestinal tract, is absorbed into the systemic circulation. It is actively transported across the lumen of the intestinal tract by way of endocytosis and transcytosis. Serotypes A and B are most efficiently transported across the intestinal lumen [27]. Similarly, wound botulism and inhalation botulism are absorbed systemically, although wound botulism may have a slower onset and progression of symptoms because of delayed absorption of the toxin [27,28]. Once botulinum toxin is in the systemic circulation, it is distributed to sites of acetylcholine-mediated neurotransmission where it causes toxicity [2,27]. The large molecular mass (150,000 d) of the botulinum toxin renders it incapable of crossing the blood-brain barrier, and as a result, all symptoms of botulism are limited to the peripheral nervous system. Although botulinum toxin is most active at the cholinergic neuromuscular junction, it is capable of inhibiting cholinergic transmission at sympathetic and parasympathetic ganglia, and at parasympathetic post-ganglionic sites [27]. However, anticholinergic symptoms tend to be mild and manifest only as a dry mouth, dilated pupils, and decreased bowel and bladder motility.

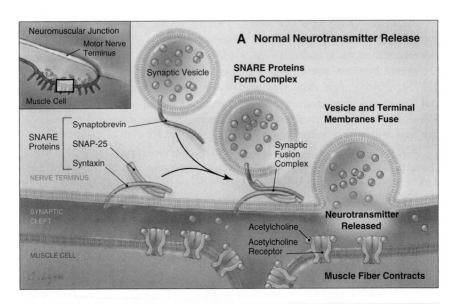

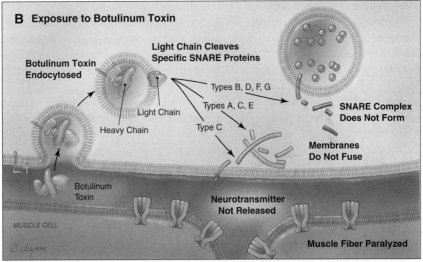

Fig. 1. Mechanism of action of botulinum toxin. (*From* Arnon SS, Schechter R, Inglesby TV, et al. Botulism toxin as a biological weapon: medical and public health management. JAMA 2001;285: 1059–70; with permission, Copyright 2001, American Medical Association. All rights reserved.)

Table 2
SNARE protein inhibition by botulinum serotype

Botulinum type	Cytosol SNARE protein inhibited
A, E	SNAP-25
B, D, F, G	Synaptobrevin
C	Syntaxin and SNAP-25

The botulinum toxin consists of a heavy and light chain that is taken up by endocytosis into the presynaptic nerve ending at the neuromuscular junction (Fig. 1) [1,27]. Once inside the neuron, the light chain is cleaved free from the heavy chain by reduction of a single disulfide bond, and acts as a zinc-dependent protease which can attack one or more of three SNARE proteins (soluble N-ethylmaleimide sensitive fusion protein attachment receptor) (Table 2). The SNARE protein complex is the key process that enables the vesicles in the nerve terminus, which contain acetylcholine, to fuse with the neural cell wall and be released into the synaptic cleft [1,27]. By preventing the release of acetylcholine, no muscular contraction can occur and flaccid paralysis results. Recovery from botulism occurs slowly over several months; a patient with serotype A disease recovers the slowest, as new neural tissue endplates are regenerated [7].

Clinical presentation

All adult forms of botulism manifest symptoms similarly [1,5–7]. The gastrointestinal forms may have a prodrome of nausea and vomiting within a few hours of ingesting contaminated food, often, however, it is not bothersome enough to seek medical care, and the diarrhea that occurs with other food-borne illnesses may not occur. Wound and inhalational botulism do not produce gastrointestinal symptoms. Onset of symptoms after exposure is variable, even within common source outbreaks, but with food-borne botulism, symptoms usually occur within 1 to 5 days of ingesting the contaminated food [5–8]. There is an inhibition of neuromuscular transmission that results in a flaccid paralysis, which occurs in a descending fashion. Bulbar palsies present first as paralysis of the motor functions of the cranial nerves. Initially, it affects the oculomotor muscles, progressing to facial muscle paralysis and then to muscles of mastication, swallowing, and eventually the larger muscles of the arms and legs. Ultimately, if unrecognized and untreated, the intercostals muscles and the diaphragm are compromised and respiratory insufficiency occurs. Once paralysis progresses to respiratory failure, the patient will need ventilator assisted support, potentially for several months, until the motor end-plate recovers [19,29].

In Box 1, the list of symptoms—the dozen D's—suggest an order of occurrence, and in the ideal setting, the diagnosis of botulism should be considered once three or four symptoms on the list occur.

Notably absent in the presentation are any central neurologic manifestations, or any sensory impairment. Also because botulism is not an infection with

---

Box 1. Symptoms of botulism: in order of appearance

Dry mouth
Diplopia (double vision)
Dilated pupils
Droopy eyes (ptosis)
Droopy face
Diminished gag reflex
Dysphagia (difficulty swallowing)
Dysarthria (difficulty articulating speech)
Dysphonia (difficulty phonating/whispered speech)
Difficulty lifting head
Descending paralysis
Diaphragmatic paralysis

---

clostridium, but rather is a manifestation of elaboration of botulinum toxin from its spores, fever is not part of the presenting symptoms. Even in cases of wound botulism, the wound does not always appear to have a significant inflammatory component, fever may be absent, and evidence of systemic infection, such as leucocytosis, may not be found [17–19].

Infant (intestinal) botulism presents differently from adult food-borne or wound botulism. Ninety-five percent of cases occur in children younger than 6 months old, and it rarely occurs after 1 year of age [24]. Almost all cases are caused by *C botulinum* serotypes A and B. Case reports of *C baratii*, type E, and *C butyricum,* type F, have occurred [9,24]. Epidemiologic investigation initially linked it to infants being given raw honey, but since most cases occur without an infant being fed honey, the pathogenesis is more likely linked to immature intestinal flora that enables the clostridium spores to colonize the bowel, germinate, and elaborate the toxin [24,25]. Both the toxin and the bacteria can be obtained from fecal samples, although a saline enema may be needed to obtain a sample. Symptoms begin with bulbar weakness such as a poor suck, and inability to hold the head upright [22]. Constipation is a prominent complaint of parents of an infant suffering from infant botulism [22,23]. This non-specific presentation often causes misdiagnosis early in the natural course of the disease. As infant botulism progresses, a more generalized muscle weakness occurs; a hypotonic floppy baby, a weak hoarse cry, and ptosis may be noted [22]. Most cases do not progress to respiratory failure; however, it has been speculated that missed cases are responsible for possible sudden infant death syndrome (SIDS) deaths [24]. Once the diagnosis is considered, hospitalization in a pediatric intensive care setting is required, because secondary complications such as pneumonia and sepsis can occur [22].

Inhalational botulism has only been described in humans after an unintentional laboratory exposure [3]. Three days after performing an autopsy on a lab animal that died of botulism, 3 technicians developed tightness in the throat, difficulty swallowing and symptoms characterized as a cold without a fever [1,3]. They developed ocular paresis, rotatory nystagmus, dilated pupils, dysarthria, ataxia, and generalized weakness. All recovered within 2 weeks with antitoxin treatment [3]. If a terrorist attack were to occur using inhaled toxin, there would likely be an irritant upper airway prodrome with the initial contact, followed by a variable onset of different degrees of paralysis in exposed victims. By three days post exposure, those maximally affected might present to a variety of out-patient and emergency department sites with the classic syndrome of descending bulbar palsies. The issue which makes this scenario most worrisome is that delayed diagnosis in a large number of patients, and the limited availability of the anti-toxin, would lead to a significant number of ventilator dependent victims immobilizing ICU care for months.

Differential diagnosis

Although a long list of neurologic and metabolic causes for motor neuropathies is frequently considered and cited in review articles [2,30], only two important diagnoses seem to be made in lieu of botulism, and accordingly delay treatment [7,11]. Myasthenia gravis is frequently considered in new onset of bulbar palsies without sensory findings, especially when isolated bilateral ptosis is the presenting complaint. In fact, the edrophonium challenge test, thought to be specific for myasthenia, may be equivocally positive in some botulism cases owing to its subjective interpretation [11,19]. The other often considered diagnosis is the Miller-Fisher variant of the Guillain-Barre syndrome. This is an

Table 3
Natural paralytic toxins which could be used as bioterrorist agents

Curare	*Strychnos toxifera*
Coral snake venom	*Micrurus fulvius*
Alpha-bungarotoxins	certain elapid snakes
Sea snake venom	*Enhydrina schistose*
Kraits	Laticaudidae
Mojave rattlesnake toxin	*Crotalus scutatus scutatus*
Textilotoxin (Australian brown snake)	*Pseudonaja textilis*
Taipoxin (Australian Taipan)	*Oxyuranus scutatus scutellatus*
Notexin (Australian tiger snake)	*Notechis scutatus scutatus*
Saxitoxin	*Gonyaulax* species
Tetrodotoxin (puffer fish)	*Fugu* species
Tarichotoxin (Newt)	*Taricha torosa*
Batrachotoxin (Columbia poison dart frog)	*Phyllobates terribilis*
Homobatrachotoxin (New Guinea Pitohui bird)	
Maculotoxin (Blue-ring octopus)	*Hapalochlaena maculosus*
Conotoxins (Cone shell)	*Conus geographus*
Gelsemine (Carolina yellow Jessamine)	*Gelsemium sempervirens*
Buckthorn	*Karwinskia humboldtiana*

exceedingly rare disorder, usually has a viral prodrome with fever, and the patient would likely initially present with ataxia [31]. Even if the Miller-Fisher variant of the Guillain-Barre syndrome is considered in the differential diagnosis, treatment for the more common botulism should be started, as time to treatment is critical for botulism.

Hypokalemic periodic paralysis and tick paralysis, two other common causes of symmetric myopathies, predominantly affect the proximal large muscles rather than cranial nerves. Most other central neurologic lesions, such as strokes, tumors, and trauma, present with unilateral findings, and some degree of central symptoms such as altered level of consciousness.

However, with multiple victims, such as in a terrorist event, the differential should include other paralytic toxins, which potentially could be derived from natural sources, such as those in Table 3.

Decontamination

Standard decontamination procedures can be used following a weaponized aerosol dispersment of suspected botulinum toxin. Because this is not an infection with clostridium, there is no risk of contagion or person-to-person transmission, and once in the hospital, the patient requires no special isolation. However, children with infant botulism may excrete the organism in their stool for several weeks, even after apparent recovery. These infants should not be placed in a setting where the organism could be passed to other infants by way of fecal contamination of toys or other fomites [22,24].

Diagnostic studies

A high clinical suspicion based on the motor exam, should be all that is needed for the treating physician to request the release of botulism antitoxin from the CDC. A young person presenting with ocular muscle findings who has not suffered a cerebral vascular accident is most likely to have botulism (Table 4) [32]. Notably absent in the clinical assessment is any change in mental status,

Table 4
The motor exam for Bulbar palsies

CN III	Can't move eyes left and right, lids droop
CN IV	Can't look downward symmetrically
CN V	Can't bite down
CN VI	Can't look outward
CN VII	Can't close eyes against force, purse lips, or smile
CN IX	Stylopharyngeus muscle only
CN X	Diminished gag reflex and difficulty swallowing & saying "Ah"
CN XI	Diminished strength trapezius and sternocleidomastoid
CN XII	Difficulty moving tongue side-to-side

sensory findings, tremor or motor hyperactivity, fever, leucocytosis, or electrolyte abnormalities.

An assessment of impending respiratory failure should include pulmonary vital capacity, which should be assessed early and repeated frequently [29]. Adjunct monitoring with end-tidal CO_2 levels may also be a vital clue to respiratory compromise.

Depending on the suspected site of entry, samples of stool, gastric content, serum, wound aspirates, or sputum may be sent in anaerobic transport media for culture of *Clostridium* species [2]. The samples ideally should be obtained before treatment with antitoxin. In the constipated infant botulism patient, a gentle saline enema may be needed to obtain a stool sample [24]. Early growth in the anaerobic culture media of the typical gram-positive bacillus suggests a clostridial species, especially if they have oval shaped subterminal spores and beta-hemolytic activity [2]. Specimens should be handled with Biosafety Level-2 containment in the microbiology laboratory [2].

Serum, stool, and suspected contaminated foods can be sent to the health department or the CDC for a mouse bioassay. If a bioterrorist event were to occur, contaminated surface swabs should also be sent for a mouse bioassay or an ELISA test [33]. The mouse bioassay is the most widely used test by health departments [2]. Although crude in its design, it is considered to be the most sensitive test for the diagnosis of botulism. Either serum or a biologic fluid supernatant is injected intraperitoneally into two sets of mice; one set pretreated with botulinum antitoxin and a control group [33]. In a positive test, the mice with the antitoxin pretreatment all live, and the untreated mice all die. A definitive result may take as long as 4 days [33]. Because there is a long turnaround time on this assay (not counting additional delays in transport to an appropriate lab), the patient should be treated on the basis of clinical suspicion rather than waiting for the assay results, which are used only to confirm and serotype the botulinum toxin involved [33]. The ELISA test is not available outside of research facilities, but has a shorter turnaround time and may be as sensitive as the mouse assay for detection of the botulinum toxin [33].

While awaiting the delivery of antitoxin, other ancillary tests may be helpful to eliminate other diagnostic possibilities. A complete set of electrolytes should help exclude potassium and magnesium disorders. A head CT scan should help eliminate central nervous system tumor or bleed, although an MRI would be necessary to exclude a brainstem lesion. A lumbar puncture can be obtained if infectious or post-infectious etiologies are considered, and an elevated cerebral spinal fluid protein suggests the Miller-Fisher variant of the Guillain-Barre syndrome [31]. If myasthenia gravis is considered, the edrophonium (Tensilon) challenge test may be administered: a saline injection is given, and the degree of upward gaze fatigability is timed, and then repeated after slow injection of edrophonium. If ptosis unequivocally improves, myasthenia gravis may be considered, but false-positive tests have been reported in cases of botulism [7,12].

Other adjuncts, such as electromyography, are best reserved until after treatment with antitoxin. Botulism causes brief small amplitude motor potentials on repetitive nerve stimulation at 20 to 50 Hz, with an incremental response to repetitive stimulation [20,34].

Treatment

As early as possible, based on history and physical exam, the treating physician should contact their local or state health department to report a suspected case of botulism. The physician should also seek assistance in acquiring the antitoxin from its cached quarantine sites at large hub airports in the United States. There are often delays and a direct call to CDC Assistance (770-488-7100) will expedite the release of the antitoxin. Some additional stores of the antitoxin may be available where frequent cases occur and distances to transport the antitoxin are great. These can be released only by decision of a state health department.

The trivalent antitoxin (against serotypes A, B, E) is the mainstay of treatment in the United States [1,35]. It contains 7500 international units (IU) type A, 5500 IU type B, and 8500 IU type E antitoxins [30,35,36]. In some areas of the country, a bivalent antitoxin against only A and B serotypes is used [10], and in Alaska and Canada, a monovalent type E antitoxin is available. A specific monovalent antitoxin against serotype F is also produced. The critical point is that administration of the antitoxin does not reverse the course of the disease, only halts its progression. It is critical to administer the antitoxin early, before respiratory insufficiency occurs, which may save the patient a prolonged course on a ventilator [29,36].

Current dosing recommendations for the trivalent antitoxin are to give a single vial diluted 1:10 in normal saline intravenously over 30 to 60 minutes [35]. Previously treatment regimens have called for both intravenous and intramuscular injections, or have included multiple vials. Because antitoxin is a horse-derived immunoglobin, the risk of allergic reactions must be appreciated. The only review citing the relative risk of allergic phenomena is an 11-year review (from 1967 to 1977) in 268 patients [37]. The skin test was administered to 151 patients; it was positive in only 9 patients, however, 2 of these patients who did not subsequently receive the recommended desensitization procedure, had anaphylaxis. Of the 142 patients who had a negative skin test, 1 had anaphylaxis and 3 had utricaria. Another 117 patients did not receive the skin test but were treated with the antitoxin and 3 of these had utricaria [37]. Five patients in each of these two groups had serum sickness. Overall, anaphylaxis occurred in 5 patients (1.9%) and was not fatal in any of them. Utricaria occurred in 7 patients (2.6%), and delayed onset serum sickness occurred in 10 (3.7%) patients; there was an overall hypersensitity rate of 9% for any type of reaction [37]. It must be noted, however, that 228 patients (85%) received more than 1 vial of antitoxin, which was the common treatment regimen at the time [37]. By comparison, the hypersensitivity rate for equine snake antivenom is 23%, which is administered far more frequently [35].

It is now known that adequate serum levels of the antitoxin for all three serotypical forms of the disease are achieved with a single vial of the trivalent antitoxin [38]. Additionally, the risk of anaphylactoid reactions can be diminished by slow administration of a dilute product. However, the package insert advises a skin test with the horse serum supplied in the package. Any decision to give the skin test must weigh the risk and benefits carefully. If the patient has had progressive paralysis, the earlier the antitoxin is given, the more likely progression can be stopped. Furthermore, neither a positive nor a negative skin test is specific to predicting nor excluding an acute allergic reaction, and because allergic reactions are rarely fatal, and time is of the essence, the risk-benefit analysis more than likely weighs in favor of giving the vial, diluted and slowly without the skin test first. Factors that weigh in favor of the skin test would be patients with: (1) an allergy history to multiple medications, (2) a prior episode of anaphylaxis from any cause, or (3) previously administered equine antitoxins (such as snake or spider antivenoms). A positive skin test would warrant pretreatment with antihistamines and steroids, and an epinephrine infusion and appropriate emergency airway equipment should be ready at the bedside to treat anaphylaxis should it occur. Given the severe consequences of delaying treatment, even in this latter scenario, it may be warranted to pretreat the patient with a history of allergies using antihistamines and steroids and then initiate the slow administration of the diluted antitoxin. Full resuscitation equipment and drugs should be immediately available in this situation.

Infant botulism cases should be treated with Human Botulism Immune Globulin that is only available through the California State Health Department (510-540-2646). This product is derived from human plasmapheresis donors who have received at least five doses of the pentavalent toxoid vaccine [24,39]. Because this is a pentavalent immune globulin against serotypes A, B, C, D, and E, it does not cover the rare occurrence of serotype F disease [39]. This product has a long biologic half-life and a greatly decreased risk of hypersensitivity reactions. It could potentially be used for adults who had an early and severe anaphylactoid reaction to the trivalent antitoxin, which would prevent a full dose from being administered [2].

The US Army has heptavalent (A–G) antitoxin that contains 4000 IU of antitoxin for types A, B, C, E, and F, and 500 IU antitoxin for serotypes D and G [1,9,40]. It is indicated for all non-A, B, E serotypes, although by the time serotype information is obtained, several days and the appropriate window of opportunity for treatment would have passed. It is sometimes referred to as a despeciated product, but it is an equine- derived immunoglobin, which has been cleaved by pepsin, thereby removing the antigenic Fc component and leaving the dual binding $F(ab')_2$ botulism immune globulin fragments [40]. This product has been used in an outbreak of type E food-borne botulism in Egypt in 1991 [40]. Of the 50 patients who received this heptavalent product, 1 developed serum sickness, and 9 had mild hypersensitivity reactions, although the data were collected retrospectively and through telephone interviews, using interpreters, relying on patient recollection of adverse events [40]. A skin test is advised for use of this product as well. The dose is a single vial diluted 1:10 in normal saline and administered over 40 to 60 minutes [40]. Similar caveats to those noted above regarding skin testing before antitoxin use should be considered with this product.

In a bioterrorist event, it may become necessary to prophylactically immunize designated individuals. A pentavalent vaccine, which has been in use for over 30 years, may be distributed by the CDC [39]. It is currently used as pretreatment for laboratory workers who may be exposed to botulism, and annual boosters are required [39]. The pentavalent vaccine is active against serotypes A, B, C, D, and E.

Adjuncts to treatment of the botulism patient include all the special features of caring for any patient with severe neurologic impairment without cognitive impairment. Early in the course, a means of communication should be established through whatever limited body movements the patient may still have. A limited group of nurses who are in tune with the patient's mode of communication might ease the frustration and depression these patients experience. Frequent inquiries as to pain and discomfort caused by body position are important. Anecdotal experience suggests that patients may have debilitating headaches that go unnoticed. Although reverse Trendelenberg position to 20 or 25 degrees has been advocated in patients not requiring intubation, the more important adjunct is frequent measuring of vital capacity in these individuals to see if intubation is required [1,29].

Once paralysis occurs, a collaborative effort by nurses, physical therapists, and respiratory therapists is needed to try to prevent the risks of infection, ventilator mishaps, and nutritional depletion that these patients experience. In one early series, a surprising number of deaths were caused by ventilator malfunctions that went unrecognized [36]. Nosocomial pneumonia, urospesis, skin breakdown and decubitus ulcer infections, and stoma infections of tracheostomies are common once the patient becomes ventilator dependent. The anticholinergic effect of the botulinum toxin may also contribute to bladder atony and thick viscid mucus secretions [8]. Muscle wasting and nutritional depletion will ultimately be impediments to weaning from the ventilator. Daily physical therapy of all paralyzed muscle groups will aid the patients rehabilitation. Frequent turning of the patient to prevent skin breakdown and pressure effects of immobilization is also important.

Prognosis

Delay to administering the antitoxin is the most important factor that affects clinical course and outcome. In one study, mortality was 10% in patients who received the antitoxin within 24 hours of onset of symptoms; 15% when it was administered later than 24 hours; and 46% when not given at all [36]. However, 4 four out of the 19 deaths in this series occurred because of ventilator malfunction or accidental extubation. The fatality rate in those over 60 years of age was twice that of those patients younger than 60 years [36].

The more rapid the onset of paralysis, the more likely intubation was needed [30]. Type A and E patients typically have a faster onsets than type B. In a review of CDC cases in 1999 and 2000, 83% of type A exposures required intubation, and only 33% of each type B and E required intubation [5,30]. In another study, the mean time on a ventilator was 58 days for serotype A cases and 26 days for serotype B cases [7]. Ventilator dependence can last as long as 142 days [8].

When there is an outbreak of botulism, the index case is usually most severely affected, and may be misdiagnosed, which causes delayed treatment [12]. Once the clinical suspicion is raised in outbreaks, subsequent cases uniformly do better [19]. It is difficult to compare outcomes between studies that have spanned many decades. Substantial improvements in critical care have reduced the mortality significantly if the disease is recognized and treated appropriately. One group, which studied long-term follow-up, indicated normal pulmonary function is regained, but diminished respiratory muscle function and easy fatigability may persist in some patients at 2 years after recovery [29,41].

Prevention

Heating above 121°C, or refrigeration below 4°C inhibits clostridial growth. To prevent spore formation, the addition of acidifying agents (eg, citric acid) is recommended for canning most vegetables. Preserving vegetables under garlic oil without canning has been identified as a particular risk factor for food-borne disease [11]. However, spores are dormant and may survive inadequate canning and vacuum procedures. The spores can withstand heating to 100°C for hours [35], but heating to 121°C under 15 to 20 lb/in² pressure for 20 minutes destroys them [5]. Interestingly, type E toxin may be resistant to freezing and may elaborate toxin during thawing of preserved marine animals above 5°C [42]. Additionally, since type E is not saccharolytic, foods contaminated with this serotype do not look or smell abnormal [42]. Once canned food is open for consumption, the botulinum toxin is destroyed by heating to 80°C for 30 minutes, or to 100°C for 10 minutes [35].

Summary

Botulinum toxin is the most lethal substance known. Six modes of disease have been recognized: (1) food-borne botulism from eating foods contaminated with *C botulinum*, (2) wound botulism from wounds harboring *C botulinum*, (3) infant (intestinal) botulism from intestinal overgrowth of *C botulinum* in children less than 1 year of age, (4) "undetermined" botulism from intestinal overgrowth of *C botulinum* in adults with surgically altered gastrointestinal tracts, (5) inadvertent (injection-related) botulism from accidental injection of Botox, and (6) inhalational botulism from aerosol exposure to botulinum toxin, as might occur in a terrorist release. Recognition of the clinical presentation characterized by bulbar palsies and descending paralysis in the absence of sensory or central nervous systems symptoms is key to making an early diagnosis. Current treatment is to administer the trivalent antitoxin against types A, B, E for adult forms, and human-derived Botulism Immune Globulin for infant botulism. A preventive pentavalent toxoid vaccine exists but must be given before exposure. Prolonged ventilator support may be required in patients with advanced paralysis.

References

[1] Arnon SS, Schechter R, Inglesby TV, et al. Botulism toxin as a biological weapon: medical and public health management. JAMA 2001;285:1059–70.

[2] Caya JG, Agni R, Miller JE. *Clostridium botulinum* and the clinical laboratorian: a detailed review, including biologic warfare ramifications of Botulinum toxin. Arch Path Lab Med 2004; 128:653–62.

[3] Middlebrook JL, Franz DR. Botulinum toxins. In: Sidell FR, Takafuji ET, Franz DR, editors. Medical aspects of chemical and biological warfare. Washington (DC): Office of the Surgeon General, Dept of the Army; 1997. p. 643–54.

[4] Zilinskas RA. Iraq's biological weapons: the past as future? JAMA 1997;278:418–24.

[5] Sobel J, Tucker N, Sulka A, et al. Food borne botulism in the United States, 1990–2000. Emerg Infect Dis 2004;10:1606–11.

[6] Shapiro RL, Hatheway C, Swerdlow DL. Botulism in the United States: a clinical and epidemiologic review. Ann Intern Med 1998;129:221–8.

[7] Hughes JM, Blumenthal JR, Merson MH, et al. Clinical features of types A and B food-borne botulism. Ann Intern Med 1981;95:442–5.

[8] Barrett DH. Endemic food-borne botulism: clinical experience, 1973–1986 at Alaska Native Medical Center. Alaska Med 1991;33:101–8.

[9] Schechter R, Arnon SS. Where Marco Polo meets Meckel: type E botulism from *Clostridium butyricum*. Clin Infect Dis 1999;29:1388–93.

[10] Richardson WH, Frei SS, Williams SR. Case of type F botulism in southern California. J Toxicol Clin Toxicol 2004;42:383–7.

[11] St. Louis ME, Peck SHS, Bowering D, et al. Botulism from chopped garlic: delayed recognition of a major outbreak. Ann Intern Med 1988;108:363–8.

[12] Angulo FJ, Getz J, Taylor JP, et al. A large outbreak of botulism: the hazardous baked potato. J Infect Dis 1998;178:172–7.

[13] Merson MH, Hughes JM, Dowell VR, et al. Current trends in botulism in the United States. JAMA 1974;229:1305–8.

[14] Merson MH, Dowell VR. Epidemiologic, clinical, and laboratory aspects of wound botulism. New Eng J Med 1973;289:1005–10.

[15] Keller MA, Miller VH, Berkowitz CD, et al. Wound botulism in pediatrics. Am J Dis Child 1982;136:320–2.

[16] Burningham MD, Walter FG, Mechem C, et al. Wound botulism. Ann Emerg Med 1994; 24:1184–7.

[17] Werner SB, Passaro D, McGee J, et al. Wound botulism in California, 1951–1998: recent epidemic in heroin injectors. Clin Infect Dis 2000;31:1018–24.

[18] Passaro DJ, Werner SB, McGee J, et al. Wound botulism associated with black tar heroin among injecting drug users. JAMA 1996;279:859–63.

[19] Horowitz BZ, Swensen E. Wound botulism associated with back tar heroin. JAMA 1998;280: 1479–80.

[20] Maselli RA, Ellis W, Mandler RN, et al. Cluster of wound botulism in California: clinical, electrophysiologic and pathologic study. Muscle Nerve 1997;20:1284–95.

[21] Spitters C, Moran J, Kruse D, et al. Wound botulism among black tar heroin users – Washington, 2003. MMWR 2003;52:885–6.

[22] Arnon SS, Midura TF, Clay SA, et al. Infant botulism: epidemiological, clinical, and laboratory aspects. JAMA 1977;237:1946–51.

[23] Reddy V, Balter S, Weiss D, et al. Infant botulism – New York City, 2001–2002. MMWR 2003; 52:21–4.

[24] Arnon SS. Infant botulism. In: Rudolph AM, Hoffman JIE, Rudolph CD, editors. Rudolph's Pediatrics. 20th edition. New York: Appleton & Lange; 1996. p. 555–8.

[25] Arnon SS, Midura TF, Damus K, et al. Honey and other environmental risk factors for infant botulism. J Pediatr 1979;94:331–6.

[26] Bakheit AMO, Ward CD, McLellan DL. Generalized botulism-like syndrome after intramuscular injections of botulism type A: a report of two cases. J Neurol Neurosurg Psych 1997;62:198.

[27] Simpson LL. Identification of the major steps in botulinum toxin action. Annu Rev Pharmacol Toxicol 2004;44:167–93.

[28] Montecucco C, Schiavo G. Mechanism of action of tetanus and botulinum neurotoxins. Mole Micro 1994;13:1–8.

[29] Wilcox PG, Andolfatto G, Fairbarn MS, et al. Long-term follow-up of symptoms, pulmonary function, respiratory muscle strength, and exercise performance after botulism. Am Rev Respir Dis 1989;139:157–63.

[30] Woodruff BA, Griffin PM, McCroskey LM, et al. Clinical and laboratory comparison of botulism from toxin types A, B, and E in the United States, 1975–1988. J Infect Dis 1992; 166:1281–3.

[31] Koga M, Yuki N. Hirata, Antecedent symptoms in Guillain-Barre syndrome: an important indicator for clinical and serological subgroups. Acta Neurol Scand 2001;103:278–87.

[32] Terranova W, Palumbo JN, Breman JG. Ocular Findings in Botulism type B. JAMA 1979; 241:475–7.

[33] Ferreira JL, Eliasberg SJ, Edmonds P, et al. Comparison of the mouse bioassay and enzyme-linked immunosorbent assay procedures for the detection of Type A botulinal toxin in food. J Food Prot 2004;67:203–6.

[34] Cherington M. Clinical spectrum of botulism. Muscle Nerve 1998;21:701–10.

[35] Goldfrank LR. Botulinum antitoxin. In: Goldfrank's Toxicologic Emergencies. 7th edition. New York: McGraw-Hill; 2002. p. 1112–4.

[36] Tacket CO, Shandera WX, Mann JM, et al. Equine antitoxin use and other factors that predict outcome in type A food borne botulism. Am J Med 1984;76:794–8.

[37] Black RE, Gunn RA. Hypersensitivity reactions associated with botulinal antitoxin. Am J Med 1980;69:567–70.

[38] Hatheway CH, Snyder JD, Seals JE, et al. Antitoxin levels in botulism patients treated with trivalent botulism antitoxin to toxin types A, B, and E. J Infect Dis 1984;150:407–12.

[39] Metzger JR, Lewis LE. Human-derived immune globulins for the treatment of botulism. Rev Infect Dis 1979;1:689–92.

[40] Hibbs RG, Weber JT, Corwin A, et al. Experience with the use of an investigational F(ab')2 heptavalent botulism immune globulin of equine origin during an outbreak of type E botulism in Egypt. Clin Infect Dis 1996;23:337–40.

[41] Wilcox PG, Morrison NJ, Pardy RL. Recovery of the ventilatory and upper airway muscles and exercise performance after type A botulism. Chest 1990;98:620–6.

[42] Horowitz BZ. Polar poisons: did botulism doom the Franklin expedition? J Toxicol Clin Toxicol 2003;41:841–7.

ELSEVIER
SAUNDERS

CRITICAL
CARE
CLINICS

Crit Care Clin 21 (2005) 841–860

Cumulative Index 2005

Note: Page numbers of article titles are in **boldface** type.

Changing Your Address?

Make sure your subscription changes too! When you notify us of your new address, you can help make our job easier by including an exact copy of your Clinics label number with your old address (see illustration below.) This number identifies you to our computer system and will speed the processing of your address change. Please be sure this label number accompanies your old address and your corrected address—you can send an old Clinics label with your number on it or just copy it exactly and send it to the address listed below.

We appreciate your help in our attempt to give you continuous coverage. Thank you.

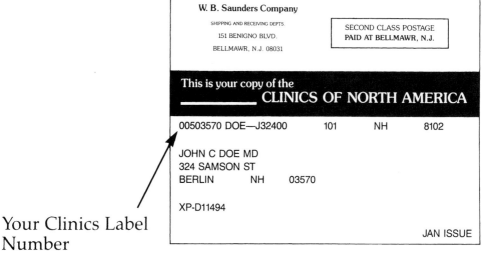

W. B. Saunders Company

SHIPPING AND RECEIVING DEPTS.

151 BENIGNO BLVD.

BELLMAWR, N.J. 08031

SECOND CLASS POSTAGE
PAID AT BELLMAWR, N.J.

This is your copy of the
_____ **CLINICS OF NORTH AMERICA**

00503570 DOE—J32400   101   NH   8102

JOHN C DOE MD
324 SAMSON ST
BERLIN   NH   03570

XP-D11494

JAN ISSUE

Your Clinics Label Number
Copy it exactly or send your label
along with your address to:
W.B. Saunders Company, Customer Service
Orlando, FL 32887-4800
Call Toll Free 1-800-654-2452

Please allow four to six weeks for delivery of new subscriptions and for processing address changes.

United States Postal Service

Statement of Ownership, Management, and Circulation

1. Publication Title									2. Publication Number										3. Filing Date
Critical Care Clinics									0	7	4	9	-	0	7	0	4			9/15/05

4. Issue Frequency	5. Number of Issues Published Annually	6. Annual Subscription Price
Jan, Apr, Jul, Oct	4	$165.00

7. Complete Mailing Address of Known Office of Publication (*Not printer*) (*Street, city, county, state, and ZIP+4*)

Elsevier, Inc.
6277 Sea Harbor Drive
Orlando, FL 32887-4800

Contact Person
Gwen C. Campbell

Telephone
215-239-3685

8. Complete Mailing Address of Headquarters or General Business Office of Publisher (*Not printer*)

Elsevier, Inc., 360 Park Avenue South, New York, NY 10010-1710

9. Full Names and Complete Mailing Addresses of Publisher, Editor, and Managing Editor (*Do not leave blank*)

Publisher (*Name and complete mailing address*)

Tim Griswold, Elsevier, Inc., 1600 John F. Kennedy Blvd. Suite 1800, Philadelphia, PA 19103-2899

Editor (*Name and complete mailing address*)

Joe Rusko, Elsevier, Inc., 1600 John F. Kennedy Blvd. Suite 1800, Philadelphia, PA 19103-2899

Managing Editor (*Name and complete mailing address*)

Heather Cullen, Elsevier, Inc., 1600 John F. Kennedy Blvd. Suite 1800, Philadelphia, PA 19103-2899

10. Owner (*Do not leave blank. If the publication is owned by a corporation, give the name and address of the corporation immediately followed by the names and addresses of all stockholders owning or holding 1 percent or more of the total amount of stock. If not owned by a corporation, give the names and addresses of the individual owners. If owned by a partnership or other unincorporated firm, give its name and address as well as those of each individual owner. If the publication is published by a nonprofit organization, give its name and address.*)

Full Name	Complete Mailing Address
Wholly owned subsidiary of	4520 East-West Highway
Reed/Elsevier, US holdings	Bethesda, MD 20814

11. Known Bondholders, Mortgagees, and Other Security Holders Owning or Holding 1 Percent or More of Total Amount of Bonds, Mortgages, or Other Securities. If none, check box ▶ ☐ None

Full Name	Complete Mailing Address
N/A	

12. Tax Status (*For completion by nonprofit organizations authorized to mail at nonprofit rates*) (*Check one*)
The purpose, function, and nonprofit status of this organization and the exempt status for federal income tax purposes:
☐ Has Not Changed During Preceding 12 Months
☐ Has Changed During Preceding 12 Months (*Publisher must submit explanation of change with this statement*)

(*See Instructions on Reverse*)

PS Form **3526**, October 1999

---

13. Publication Title	14. Issue Date for Circulation Data Below
Critical Care Clinics	JULY 2005

15.	Extent and Nature of Circulation		Average No. Copies Each Issue During Preceding 12 Months	No. Copies of Single Issue Published Nearest to Filing Date
a.	Total Number of Copies (*Net press run*)		3150	2900
b. Paid and/or Requested Circulation	(1)	Paid/Requested Outside-County Mail Subscriptions Stated on Form 3541. (*Include advertiser's proof and exchange copies*)	1589	1537
	(2)	Paid In-County Subscriptions Stated on Form 3541 (*Include advertiser's proof and exchange copies*)		
	(3)	Sales Through Dealers and Carriers, Street Vendors, Counter Sales, and Other Non-USPS Paid Distribution	477	573
	(4)	Other Classes Mailed Through the USPS		
c.	Total Paid and/or Requested Circulation (*Sum of 15b. (1), (2), (3), and (4)*)	▶	2066	2110
d. Free Distribution by Mail (*Samples, complimentary, and other free*)	(1)	Outside-County as Stated on Form 3541	95	115
	(2)	In-County as Stated on Form 3541		
	(3)	Other Classes Mailed Through the USPS		
e.	Free Distribution Outside the Mail (*Carriers or other means*)			
f.	Total Free Distribution (*Sum of 15d. and 15e.*)	▶	95	115
g.	Total Distribution (*Sum of 15c. and 15f*)	▶	2161	2225
h.	Copies not Distributed		989	675
i.	Total (*Sum of 15g. and h.*)	▶	3150	2900
j.	Percent Paid and/or Requested Circulation (*15c. divided by 15g. times 100*)		96%	95%

16. Publication of Statement of Ownership
☐ Publication required. Will be printed in the **October 2005** issue of this publication.   ☐ Publication not required

17. Signature and Title of Editor, Publisher, Business Manager, or Owner

Janet Zimmerman Date 9/15/05

Janet Zimmerman – Manager of Subscription Services

I certify that all information furnished on this form is true and complete. I understand that anyone who furnishes false or misleading information on this form or who omits material or information requested on the form may be subject to criminal sanctions (including fines and imprisonment) and/or civil sanctions (including civil penalties).

Instructions to Publishers

1. Complete and file one copy of this form with your postmaster annually on or before October 1. Keep a copy of the completed form for your records.
2. In cases where the stockholder or security holder is a trustee, include in items 10 and 11 the name of the person or corporation for whom the trustee is acting. Also include the names and addresses of individuals who are stockholders who own or hold 1 percent or more of the total amount of bonds, mortgages, or other securities of the publishing corporation. In item 11, if none, check the box. Use blank sheets if more space is required.
3. Be sure to furnish all circulation information called for in item 15. Free circulation must be shown in items 15d, e, and f.
4. Item 15h., Copies not Distributed, must include (1) newsstand copies originally stated on Form 3541, and returned to the publisher, (2) estimated returns from news agents, and (3), copies for office use, leftovers, spoiled, and all other copies not distributed.
5. If the publication had Periodicals authorization as a general or requester publication, this Statement of Ownership, Management, and Circulation must be published; it must be printed in any issue in October or, if the publication is not published during October, the first issue printed after October.
6. In item 16, indicate the date of the issue in which this Statement of Ownership will be published.
7. Item 17 must be signed.
Failure to file or publish a statement of ownership may lead to suspension of Periodicals authorization.

PS Form **3526**, October 1999 (*Reverse*)